DENTAL STATISTICS MADE EASY

Third Edition

DENTAL STATISTICS MADE EASY

Third Edition

NIGEL C. SMEETON

Centre for Research in Primary and Community Care
University of Hertfordshire, UK
and
Division of Imaging Sciences and Biomedical Engineering
King's College, London, UK

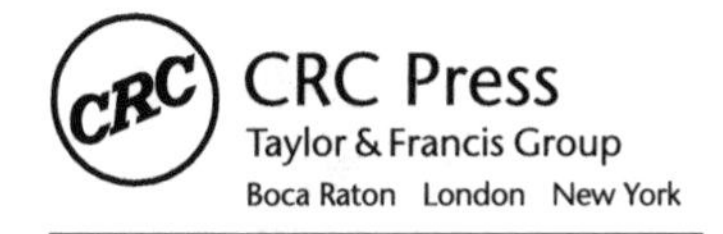

CRC Press is an imprint of the
Taylor & Francis Group, an **informa** business
A CHAPMAN & HALL BOOK

CRC Press
Taylor & Francis Group
6000 Broken Sound Parkway NW, Suite 300
Boca Raton, FL 33487-2742

Printed on acid-free paper
Version Date: 20160609

International Standard Book Number-13: 978-1-4987-7505-2 (Paperback)

Library of Congress Cataloging-in-Publication Data

Names: Smeeton, N. C., author.
Title: Dental statistics made easy / Nigel C. Smeeton.
Description: Third edition. | Boca Raton, FL : CRC Press, [2016] | Includes bibliographical references and index.
Identifiers: LCCN 2016022440| ISBN 9781498775052 (pbk. : alk. paper) | ISBN 9781498775069 (e-book) | ISBN 9781498775083 (e-book) | ISBN 9781498775076 (e-book)
Subjects: | MESH: Statistics as Topic--methods | Dental Research--methods
Classification: LCC RK52.45 | NLM WU 20.5 | DDC 617.60072/7--dc23
LC record available at https://lccn.loc.gov/2016022440

Visit the Taylor & Francis Web site at
http://www.taylorandfrancis.com

and the CRC Press Web site at
http://www.crcpress.com

Printed and bound in the United States of America by
Edwards Brothers Malloy on sustainably sourced paper

Contents

Preface to the Third Edition

My background in teaching dental statistics goes back to the early 1990s, when I became engaged in introducing the basics of study design and data analysis to undergraduate dental students at the very start of their professional training. This experience was supplemented by visits to dental practical sessions (complete with lab coat) where I was able to see first hand the collection of data such as salivary flow rates. At that time, medical students were able to choose from a range of medical statistics texts, whereas there were few introductory statistics books written specifically with dental training in mind. In addition, it was not uncommon for dental students to feel challenged by the mathematical approach then in common use.

This gap in student learning resources was initially addressed through the development of tailored course notes that included guided tutorials along with detailed solutions. In addition, students were introduced to dental journal literature through articles on major issues such as the fluoridation of public water supplies and dental health provision in areas of deprivation. The material was well received by dental students and staff alike, and it became clear that there was a need for a textbook in dental statistics which cut through the algebra and focused directly on the issues that bring dentistry and statistics together. The encouragement of my colleagues and dental students at King's College London brought about the publication of *Dental Statistics Made Easy* in 2005, with a second edition in 2012.

The needs of qualified dentists and those engaged in dental research have not been overlooked. The collection and interpretation of information is essential in, for instance, the development of new treatments, the delivery of dental care in the community, and the administration of patient records at a dental practice. This book provides an introduction to how this information is collected and analyzed, and the role that academic publication plays in the dissemination of research findings. There is an emphasis on underlying principles, illustrated by drawing from published dental studies and realistic examples rather than through recourse to algebraic formulae.

The first chapter explains why familiarity with dental statistics is important. The next chapters provide a broad overview of study design. Attention is given to the use of pilot studies, public and patient involvement in research, and ethical considerations, as well as to the common types of design and most widely used methods of sampling. The reader is then introduced to the Normal distribution, diagnostic testing, and the concept of sampling variation. Subsequent chapters cover the analysis of dental data, with an emphasis on the use of null hypotheses and the interpretation of confidence intervals (details of some of the calculations are provided in the Appendix). The book concludes with a description of how a review of the dental literature can be applied to modify everyday dental practice, followed by an account of the process involved in the development of a dental paper from the initial drafting of a report to its eventual publication in an academic journal.

This text has been written with a wide audience in mind, including dental students, qualified dentists, those engaged in dental research, and health-care professionals in general. No previous knowledge of statistics is required, and, importantly for readers who are not dentists, the illustrative examples are accessible to those involved in other areas of health care. Its style makes the book suitable not only as a class text but also for self-directed learning. The main text provides a gentle introduction to dental statistics, with exercises and solutions available for readers taking an in-depth approach. The numerous key messages allow the time-pressured dentist to benefit from a superficial reading and enable the most important principles to be located quickly. The articles used in the book, along with the associated cited and citing papers, will aid in identifying up-to-date subject-specific literature for student dissertations, library projects, and dental research.

NEW TO THIS EDITION

Some of the features of the present edition are the following:

- A new chapter on evidence-based dentistry. This material covers the "why" and "how" of systematic reviews along with a very basic introduction to meta-analysis. Emphasis is placed on sources of information, the hierarchy of research and the concept of research quality. This chapter also covers the neglected area of publications in languages other than English. An intriguing question that has received scant attention is addressed: Do dentists actually implement what they discover through evidence-based dentistry in their routine dental care?

- The selection of dental journal articles used in the examples and exercises has been broadened and updated. The perspective of the book is much more international, particularly, but not exclusively, with regard to the United States, and examples have been drawn from a range of cultures around the world.
- The assumption of independence of observations required for most basic statistical techniques has been highlighted.
- The conduct of pilot studies is explained in greater detail. In addition, the use of public and patient involvement (PPI) in research is described as funding organizations increasingly expect proposed studies to include PPI input.
- In the description of cohort studies, retrospective as well as prospective designs are discussed.
- Cluster randomized trials have been included as part of the material on randomized controlled trials.
- In the comparison of several means, a caution is given regarding the use of the Bonferroni technique.
- Illustrative examples have been modified. In part, this is to ensure that the data are appropriate for the statistical methods described. In addition, a caution has been given regarding current opinion on the benefits of water fluoridation. Increasing public concern regarding patient home to dental practice distance explains the choice of this issue for several examples.

ACKNOWLEDGMENTS

I wish to thank the many readers and reviewers who have provided detailed constructive feedback on the earlier editions, and my colleagues at the Centre for Research in Primary and Community Care, University of Hertfordshire, for their encouragement in my commitment to making statistics accessible to all. Any imperfections in the text are, of course, my responsibility.

Nigel Smeeton
August 2016

Preface to the Second Edition

This text was developed for the dental student or practitioner who wishes to discover the rationale behind the application of statistics to dentistry. Practical dental examples were employed to illustrate these concepts without the need to resort to algebraic formulae. Feedback received since its publication in 2005 has shown that readers, including some from outside the dental community, have found this book helpful as a first step on their pathway to understanding and using statistics.

The content of the original text was chosen to reflect the current key statistical issues at the time of writing. Although the importance of these core principles remains unquestioned, the range of statistical methods routinely found in the dental literature has subsequently broadened and study findings are frequently presented in greater detail than in the past. This edition covers some of the additional issues that these advances have raised, whilst retaining the original focus on the understanding of statistical concepts rather than the performance of routine calculations.

The text has been supplemented by a chapter on one-way analysis of variance. This topic forms a natural extension of the unpaired *t*-test to the case of three or more independent groups. The role of confidence intervals in the presentation of results has been given much greater emphasis and the use of confidence intervals in diagnostic testing, regression and correlation, and the analysis of observer agreement is discussed. The original chapter on non-Normally distributed data has been extended in order to introduce the use of analysis of variance and correlation in situations where the data cannot be assumed to follow a Normal distribution.

The choice of the dental journal papers used for the examples and exercises has been updated. It is intended that these papers, along with their cited references, will not only be helpful in the study of dental statistics in its own right but will also aid in locating appropriate subject-specific literature for student dissertations, library projects and dental research. Advances in technology are transforming many aspects of the research process from data entry to the way in which journals handle potential papers for publication. These developments have also been reflected in this edition.

Finally, I wish to thank the many colleagues and dental students who provided the original motivation for this book. The students engaged in the Master of Public Health course at King's College London have, by their enthusiastic feedback, aided in encouraging me to write this updated edition. Regarding the exercises, I am particularly grateful to King's College London for permitting the use of several dental undergraduate examination questions, as indicated in the text. Any imperfections in the text are, of course, my responsibility.

Nigel Smeeton
April 2012

Preface to the First Edition

Throughout my experience of teaching the basic principles of statistics to dental undergraduates and researchers, students and colleagues have remarked on the need for a textbook in dental statistics that cuts through the algebra and focuses directly on the issues that bring dentistry and statistics together. It is in this spirit that this text has been developed, drawing from the course in dental statistics at King's College, London. It is intended for the dental student or practitioner who wishes to discover the rationale behind the application of statistics to dentistry. These concepts are illustrated by practical dental examples without the reader having to contend with formulae or even mathematical symbols. To assist the reader in gaining rapid reference to specific concepts, use has been made of highlighted key points.

As for the concepts themselves, statistics is a huge field in its own right and those chosen represent what are in my view the key issues. The scope of the book is wide and covers such areas as research ethics, dealing with statistical referees and a simplified introduction to sample size calculation. Hence, basic methods of data presentation and the use of statistical techniques have been given a much less important place than in the traditional statistics text.

There are several ways open for these basic concepts to be explored more closely. The Appendix has been designed so that some of the simpler calculations can be followed through. Where the discussion shows signs that it might become technical, references to texts and journal articles have been given so that these issues can be followed further. Finally, at the end of most chapters there is a wide range of exercises. Some of these are in a multiple-choice form, whereas others require a few sentences in response. There are several longer problems based on studies published in dental journals and an extended case study around research design. All questions have been provided with solutions. For some there is a straightforward answer, for others a well-reasoned argument might be presented from more than one position; problems in research are usually of the latter kind so it is only fair to give the reader due warning.

In writing this book I wish to thank the many colleagues and dental students who have been involved in the development of the King's College dental statistics course over the years. Any imperfections in the text are, of course, totally my responsibility. I am also grateful to King's College, London, for permitting the use of several dental undergraduate examination questions, as indicated in the text.

Nigel Smeeton
December 2004

CHAPTER 1

Introduction

Dentistry is a rapidly evolving profession. Methods of patient management are under constant scrutiny and there is a wide range of views about the funding of dental care. New methods of diagnosis and treatment continue to be developed. The current rapid advances in technology will without doubt accelerate this process.

Before new methods can be considered suitable for general implementation, they need to be compared with current techniques. Such studies often yield much detailed information that has to be evaluated. For example: Is the new technique "better"? Are there any side effects? What are the cost implications? In order to resolve these questions properly, a multidisciplinary team is required that includes (for example) psychologists, sociologists, economists, and statisticians. Dental statistics plays a crucial role in the design and evaluation of such studies. Once the findings have been summarized, they need to be applied to the practice of dentistry in general. Statistical methods are essential in order to achieve this goal.

It is the responsibility of the qualified dentist to keep abreast of developments in dental practice, particularly those that are relevant to the quality of patient care. In many countries, practicing dentists are required to undertake continuing professional development (CPD) in order to remain registered. Information about dental care is more readily available to the general public than ever before (e.g., on the Internet), and some patients will ask their dentist detailed questions about their treatment. A basic knowledge of statistics can enable the dentist to become better informed about dental issues. In particular, it can assist in the following.

THE UNDERSTANDING OF PAPERS IN JOURNALS

One component of many CPD programs is the critical reading of a number of dental articles. Dentists might also need to evaluate papers on themes related to their particular specialty. Articles of general interest to dentists appear in high-circulation dental periodicals such as the *British Dental Journal* and the *Journal of the American Dental Association*. Papers of interest to a particular field of dentistry tend to appear in specialist journals such as *Community Dental Health*, the *International Journal of Paediatric Dentistry*, and the *Journal of Oral and Maxillofacial Surgery*. Occasionally, dental articles of potential interest to all clinicians are published in high-circulation medical journals such as the *British Medical Journal*, the *Journal of the American Medical Association*, and *The Lancet*. Many papers (both general and specialist) make use of statistical terms; some knowledge of statistics will therefore make it much easier to glean useful information from them. It is unwise to have blind faith in everything that is published; journal articles can contain errors and a little knowledge of dental statistics can assist in the detection of some of them.

Day-to-day clinical decisions should be based on the current evidence (this is known as evidence-based dentistry). To facilitate this process, the journal *Evidence-Based Dentistry* publishes abstracts of important advances in the practice of dentistry. Many of these summarize the results of a comprehensive search of literature databases such as MEDLINE, a continually updated source of information on articles from medical, dental, and biological journals (see Chapter 17). This relieves the busy dental practitioner of what can be a very time-consuming task.

CLINICAL AUDIT

In many dental practices, patients complete a short information sheet when they register. This usually requests the patient's name, address, gender, date of birth, current medical conditions, and medications prescribed. A dental record is created for that patient. Information regarding the condition of the patient's teeth, investigative procedures, and treatment received is added after each visit by the patient. It is good practice to audit dental records to assess (for instance) procedures performed, patient referrals, and methods of payment for care. In many countries, dental practices operate in a free market and careful financial auditing is essential.

Suppose that a new method of treatment is adopted at a dental practice. The partners will need to evaluate its success (or otherwise) from the records of patients in the practice. If the findings are in the form of numbers, the use of statistical methods is the most appropriate form of evaluation.

HEALTH SERVICES RESEARCH

Increasingly, general dental practices are being linked to dental schools for the purpose of research studies in the community. Practices can act as data-collecting centers for projects based, for instance, in a dental school. In addition, if they so wish, dentists can learn about research methods and gain assistance with the planning of their own investigations, thus becoming active researchers in their own right.

The view that few dental students or practitioners are interested in participating in research is becoming increasingly outdated. Dental practice research networks have developed into a major resource (Heasman et al. 2015) at local, regional, and national dental practice levels. Some involvement in research activities is becoming increasingly commonplace. The origin of one of the earliest general dental practice networks in the United Kingdom (UK) is described below.

Example 1.1

Kay, Ward, and Locker (2003) describe the development of a general dental practice research network in the northwest of England. Some general dental practitioners in the region were interested in participating in research in an active way beyond data collection alone. Following funding from a research and development initiative for primary dental care, a series of workshops was organized. These were aimed at developing the research skills of practitioners in areas such as literature retrieval, critical appraisal of articles, questionnaire design, applying for research funding, and data analysis. A further goal was to stimulate the practitioners' own research ideas, so that the network could undertake a research program leading to publications in refereed journals.

Fifteen dentists, each from a different practice, joined the network. The scheme was judged to be highly successful with all the aims being met, including the publication of research papers. Participant feedback highlighted a strong sense of belonging to a group, considerable personal educational development, and increased job satisfaction. Most practitioners thought that their involvement in the network would improve the standard of their patient care.

Dental practice research networks are now found worldwide. These include the National Dental Practice-Based Research Network (US), the Scottish Dental Practice Based Research Network (UK), the Dental Practice Based Research Network Japan, and the eviDent Foundation (State of Victoria, Australia).

A LITTLE HISTORY

In 1916, Henry Ford, the famous American pioneer of automobile production, declared: "History is bunk." Most health professionals would disagree; finding out about the historical development of research methods can be very instructive. A basic consideration of study design is the number of individuals involved in the project. If this is not a sufficiently large sample, important differences between groups might be missed or put down to chance; this idea will be developed in later chapters. Before the 1920s most dental research was conducted by individual dentists with limited resources. The earliest studies tended therefore to be too small to lead to definite conclusions. Little attention was given to the number of patients realistically required.

Example 1.2

Owen (1898) described a series of four cases of swallowing artificial teeth treated in the Royal Southern Hospital, Liverpool, during a six-month period (Table 1.1).

This study provides evidence that those who had their artificial teeth extracted died, whereas those for whom events took their natural course survived. However, for a series of four patients this finding could have occurred just by chance. Had a similar pattern been found with 200 or even 20 patients in each group, the results would have been much more impressive. To make a simple analogy, consider a

TABLE 1.1 Characteristics of a series of patients who swallowed their artificial teeth

Patient	*Sex*	*Age (years)*	*Action taken*	*Outcome*
1	Male	30	Removed from esophagus	Died (12 days) – septicemia
2	Male	56	Extracted from throat by forceps	Died (2 days) – syncope
3	Male	19	Allowed to pass through rectum	Survived
4	Female	35	Allowed to pass through rectum	Survived

coin that shows the head of state on one side ("head") and a design appropriate to that state on the other ("tail"). If such a coin were to be tossed twice, it would not be unusual to obtain two heads, whereas 20 heads from 20 tosses would cast grave doubt on the assumption that heads and tails are equally likely.

Readers interested in the evolution of dental research may find the landmark survey published by the US National Academy of Sciences of the literature related to dental caries to be an invaluable resource (Toverud et al. 1952). As dental research has advanced, studies have tended to become larger in order to detect small but important differences between groups or in trends over time. Today, research investigations may involve hundreds or even thousands of patients in multiple locations. This scale of research has led to the need for extensive collaboration between colleagues, dental practices, and dental hospitals within and even between different countries.

Example 1.3

The Health Behaviour in School-aged Children (HBSC) study is an international World Health Organization (WHO) initiative that involves data collection on the health and well-being, social environments, and health behaviors of young people aged 11, 13 and 15 years. Information is collected every four years from each participating country using classroom-based self-report questionnaires. The phase conducted in 2013/2014 involved 42 countries and almost 220,000 participants (Inchley et al. 2016).

Each time the survey is conducted the questions tend to follow a similar pattern. Items of particular interest to dental research that have been used at each phase, so that trends across time can be studied, include frequency of teeth brushing and soft-drink/soda consumption. The international reports display findings subdivided by age group, gender, and country. It is therefore possible to find highly specific information such as, for instance, the proportion of 11-year-old girls in France who brush their teeth more than once a day for 2013/2014 (indicated as 82%). For England, teeth brushing and dietary information is available for the phases between 1997/1998 and 2013/2014.

A FEW BASIC DEFINITIONS

Key Message 1.1: Sampling

When we conduct a study we collect information or data on a group of individuals known as a sample. The characteristics for which information is recorded are known as variables.

In Example 1.2, the sample is a group of four adult patients who swallowed their artificial teeth, and the variables are gender, age, action taken, and outcome. In Example 1.3, the overall sample is a group of almost 220,000 young people, and the variables include gender, age, and country of residence.

Qualitative variables have no numerical significance. They can be binary, having just two categories (e.g., sex: male, female); nominal, with several categories (e.g., cause of death: septicemia, syncope, did not die), or ordered (e.g., level of pain on swallowing teeth: mild, moderate, severe).

Quantitative variables are those that are measured either as whole numbers (e.g., a count of missing teeth) or are continuous (e.g., daily sugar consumption).

SAMPLES AND POPULATIONS

Although samples can provide interesting information in their own right, they are generally collected in order to make deductions about the group of people that they represent, known as the **population**. In dentistry, the population of interest is usually a group of people with a specified set of characteristics (e.g., patients registered at a particular dental practice).

Key Message 1.2: Relation of the Sample to the Population

At the start of a study the appropriate population should be identified. Once the study has been designed, the sample is then drawn from this population. Analysis of the information from the sample enables deductions to be made about the population.

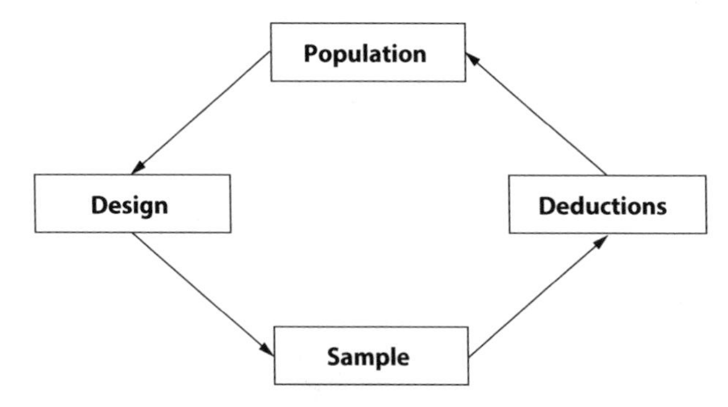

FIGURE 1.1 The cycle of research.

Ideally, samples should reflect the characteristics of the population. However, this is often not the case; for example, the proportion of females is much higher in the sample compared to the population (the practice list, say, compared to all local people). Such a sample is **biased**; this concept and its implications for research will be discussed in more detail in Chapter 2.

Future studies of a similar nature might allow for detailed information to be built up about the population. Figure 1.1 illustrates the way in which knowledge can be built up about a specific area of dental research.

TEST YOUR UNDERSTANDING

1 Using the table below, match each variable to its type.
Options:
(a) Binary
(b) Nominal
(c) Ordered
(d) Whole number quantitative
(e) Continuous quantitative

Patient number	*Gender*	*Exact age (years)*	*Number of fillings*	*Type of patient*	*Self-reported level of pain*
1	Male	33.6	1	G	Mild
2	Female	20.5	0	P	Severe
3	Female	41.9	5	D	Moderate
4	Male	49.3	3	G	Moderate
5	Female	27.4	1	G	Mild

G, government health care; P, private; D, dental insurance.

(i) Gender
(ii) Exact age
(iii) Number of fillings
(iv) Type of patient (G, P, or D)
(v) Self-reported level of pain.

2 The type of dental treatment that a patient receives could be classified as either a nominal or an ordered variable. Explain using an example why this is the case.
3 Describe using examples two ways in which the knowledge of statistical procedures can be useful to the dental practitioner.
4 If you are a qualified dentist, reflect on how statistical ideas might be relevant to your own CPD. You might find it illuminating to repeat the exercise after having worked through this text!

CHAPTER 2

Planning a Study

INTRODUCTION

As with any worthwhile endeavor, embarking on the study of an issue related to dentistry can have considerable resource implications in terms of both time and money. Dedicated time will need to be put aside by the dentist, in terms of learning about research techniques that may be unfamiliar. In addition, time might need to be committed to meeting with other dentists and non-clinical experts about the study design, collaboration with colleagues in the data collection, guidance in the data analysis, and dissemination of the results. There is a cost involved in terms of the income that the dentist might otherwise have generated by treating patients (Kay, Ward, and Locker 2003). For a larger study additional clerical staff might need to be employed to deal with, for instance, the paperwork, telephone calls, and data input generated by the study. Are research studies really necessary?

One compelling argument for conducting this type of study is that casual appearances can be deceptive. Day-to-day impressions cannot be relied upon. A dentist may notice that patients who admit to consuming large quantities of fizzy drinks seem to need more fillings. This view might develop because the dentist is more likely to ask patients about their diet if they require a considerable amount of dental work to be done. A dental inspection that reveals no problems with a patient's teeth might not generate much conversation about dental issues. Furthermore, the dentist might assume that the patient has a healthy diet and cleans his teeth regularly. The working of the human mind is generally such that particularly advanced cases of dental decay will remain in the memory long after the details of patients with few dental problems have been forgotten. The memory recall of both the dentist and the patient can be far from perfect. If there is a genuine association between the consumption of fizzy drinks and the need for fillings, this does not necessarily imply that there is a cause and effect relationship between diet and dental health. Other associated factors might be of more relevance. For instance, patients who consume many fizzy drinks might also have a more dismissive attitude toward their dental health. Hence they might take less effort in looking after their teeth; for example, brushing their teeth less frequently and thoroughly, visiting the dentist only when in pain, and neglecting to use mouthwash for their gums.

Another strong reason for the implementation of research studies involving individual patients is that it is necessary to investigate individuals in order to make deductions about individuals. Information about geographical regions is sometimes readily available in official documents, in which case it is straightforward to access relationships at that level without recourse to personal research (Murray, Vernazza, and Holmes 2015). However, a relationship that is observed when geographical areas (e.g., towns) form the units of interest might not have been produced as a result of the same relationship existing at the level of the individual. This assumption of the existence of a relationship for individuals purely because it occurs at a regional level can lead to what is known as the **ecological fallacy**. For instance, in a comparison of regions, the average sugar consumption per year may be associated with the proportion of individuals without teeth. However, it cannot immediately be concluded that sugar consumption influences an individual's chances of losing all his or her teeth. It might be that the regions with greatest levels of sugar consumption also have high proportions of elderly people, who tend to have fewer natural teeth. The issue might be complicated by a possible variation in the consumption of alternative sweeteners between regions.

If more needs to be discovered about a dentist's own practice, it can be misleading to apply findings produced from studies conducted elsewhere. The patients on the dentist's register might have quite different characteristics in terms of residential circumstances, age structure, ethnicity, and socioeconomic levels. The dental needs of a community are influenced by these variables, so information about the dentist's specific population of interest (often the complete practice list) is required.

STAGES OF A STUDY

For a study to be effective and yield reliable results, the research needs to be well planned. The quality of the study design is important whether the investigation is a small undergraduate student project or a large-scale trial involving research teams based in different parts of the world. Although it might be tempting to overlook aspects of the later stages of the investigation such as data analysis and interpretation, these should be taken into account at the design stage. The use of sophisticated statistical methods in the data analysis is rarely able to correct for design flaws overlooked in a hastily conducted study. Where feasible, members of the population under consideration should have an input into the study design and conduct.

Each of the main stages of a study will be considered below. The list is not exhaustive but points out important milestones along the way.

State the Problem

The issue of interest needs to be formulated in terms of a question that can be investigated (e.g., Is periodontal disease related to smoking?). However, in order for the project to be feasible it will need to be focused on a particular group (e.g., Is gingivitis in adults living in Los Angeles exacerbated by smoking?).

> **Key Message 2.1: Research Question**
>
> The question(s) to be answered should be formulated before the study is carried out. If it is possible to answer several questions at the same time without overcomplicating the design, the limited time and money available will be used to greater effect.

Conduct a Literature Review

Another research team may have solved the problem already! Check the relevant literature; in any case, published articles will indicate how research work of a similar nature has developed. Papers are also useful for learning from the mistakes and successes of others without having to find out the hard way.

Decide How the Data are to be Obtained

For some studies, information is obtained directly from individuals through questionnaires, face-to-face interviews, and dental examinations. Other studies involve the use of dental records. Information might be obtained from dental practices or hospitals. There is a wide range of sampling techniques available (see Chapter 4) and a method suitable for the particular study should be chosen.

Key Message 2.2: Objective and Subjective Measures

Most studies use a combination of objective and subjective measures. Objective information, such as the number of fillings in a patient's mouth, is not influenced by the personal views of the dentist making the inspection. On the other hand, subjective information such as a patient's assessment of his or her degree of pain during treatment can be influenced by factors such as pain threshold and expectations of the likely level of pain prior to the procedure.

The size of the sample to be collected is largely dictated by the time and money available for the research. Thought should be given at this stage about how the project will be funded; additional resources from grant-awarding bodies are likely to be required beyond those personally available to the dentists involved (see p. 18).

Whatever the likely source of funding, the minimum number of patients required to demonstrate a particular important clinical finding should be stated in advance. Failure to detect an important finding because too small a sample is chosen is a waste of resources and ethically wrong (see Chapter 6). On this basis, an estimate should be made of the likely sample size required for a reasonable chance of discovering useful findings. Such estimates, obtained from what are known as sample-size calculations, are considered in greater detail in Chapter 16. If the estimate for the sample-size requirement is larger than that envisaged in initial planning discussions, an extension of the period of data collection or the recruitment of other dental practitioners to the study might be the answer.

Key Message 2.3: Unit of Data

The unit of data analysis is the basic element of data collected for the sample. It is the number of these units that is estimated in the sample-size calculation. In the analysis, individual observations come from each unit.

In designing the data collection, the unit of data should be made clear. In many studies, such as those that involve satisfaction questionnaires completed by the patient, it is the individual. Studies involving clinical examination might take the tooth as the unit of data. Those that consider the characteristics of the dental practice building (e.g., ease of access for disabled patients) would take the dental practice as the unit of data.

Obtain Ethical Approval

In most parts of the world, studies that involve the recruitment of patients require ethical approval from the relevant hospitals and local health authorities before they can proceed. A grant-awarding body will have a similar requirement for proposals that it receives for possible funding. By this stage in the planning, the fundamental issues in the study design should have been addressed. Ideally, this process should include meetings with representatives of the individuals involved in order to obtain patient or client perspectives. These meetings should highlight glaring problems such as poorly worded questionnaire items. Involvement with members of the public should take place before ethical approval is sought, as this may increase the likelihood of a positive decision.

Ethical approval is generally obtained by using the ethical committee's application form and attaching a copy of the study proposal. More than one local research ethics committee (LREC) may have to be involved depending, for example, on the nature of the study and the geographical distribution of the practices concerned.

This can be problematic if the ethical committees involved reach conflicting decisions. Multicenter research ethics committees (MRECs) have been established to enable potential studies involving several centers to be considered by just one committee. This avoids the difficulties created by conflicting ethical committee decisions and makes more efficient use of committee time.

In the UK, application for permissions and approvals for research in health and social care has been simplified through the introduction of the Integrated Research Application System (IRAS). This enables researchers to provide the relevant information from their project proposal using one form. This information is then accessed by the appropriate review bodies, avoiding the submission of a separate application to each reviewing committee.

Members of ethical committees are chosen from fields relevant to human medical research, and can include clinicians and biological scientists, a legal expert, a professional ethicist and a statistician. Many ethical committees involve lay representatives from the local community.

For most ethical committees, straightforward cases are dealt with by correspondence, the committee deciding on applications at regularly held meetings. The usual decisions are acceptance, acceptance subject to modifications required by the committee, or rejection. More complicated proposals and those for which the committee members are unwilling to make an immediate decision by correspondence alone can involve one or more of the applicants attending a meeting to be questioned in person.

Conduct a Pilot Study

Before the main study is conducted, it is prudent to carry out the procedures involved with a relatively small series of individuals, a process described as conducting a pilot or feasibility study (Lancaster, Dodd, and Williamson 2004, Thabane et al. 2010). This phase is often viewed as less important than the main study, for instance, as an opportunity for a student project (Thabane et al. 2010). In order to correct this misconception, it is important that clear objectives are defined. These should include: estimating an appropriate sample size for the main study; testing of questionnaires; assessing the practicalities of recruitment and consent; checking whether the initial estimates of the costs involved in terms of time and money are realistic; ascertaining the acceptability of any interventions; and, if unclear, making a final decision on the choice of the main outcome to be studied (Lancaster, Dodd, and Williamson 2004).

Findings from pilot studies should be descriptive. An in-depth statistical assessment of the results should be avoided as the identification of important findings at the pilot stage offers the temptation to dispense with the main study altogether. Continuing with the main study enables confirmation or rejection of encouraging findings from a pilot study and provides deeper insight into any relationships between the study variables.

There is no convention regarding an appropriate sample size for pilot studies. A minimum of 30 participants has been suggested (Lancaster, Dodd, and Williamson 2004), although if suitable individuals are difficult to identify and/or recruit this guideline can be challenging. In terms of outliers, a sample of 30 observations is able to give an impression of what might be regarded as "typical."

In project development, external pilot studies are generally preferred. In this situation, the information collected during the pilot study is not incorporated into the data used for the main study analyses. The alternative, an internal pilot study, makes use of the pilot data in the final analyses. This approach is likely to introduce bias where modifications have been made to the study design following the pilot stage.

Carry out the Main Study

At this stage, equipment specifically required for the study should be purchased and any additional members of staff needed should be recruited. Data recording sheets and, if required, final versions of questionnaires, should be produced. The day-to-day routines involved in the study need to be set in motion. Staff training may be required. For instance, in a practice-based study involving patient-completed questionnaires, receptionists may need to be reminded to give patients a questionnaire as they arrive, collect completed questionnaires before they leave, and answer their queries about the study. If a patient prefers to complete the questionnaire at home, a postage paid envelope should be provided. Training individuals in data collection is particularly worthwhile if the information to be collected has a subjective element. For instance, some studies involve the assessment of interobserver agreement (see Chapter 14) and only commence in earnest once this is satisfactory.

The accuracy of the data sets produced by a research study is crucial for the analysis. If the data are unreliable the results are, at best, likely to be misleading. Usually, data are collected during face-to-face interviews or recorded on questionnaires. During interviews, the information could be taken down inaccurately. Items of a questionnaire could inadvertently be answered differently from the respondent's intention. With long questionnaires, a whole sheet might be overlooked. It is generally impractical to check answers to particular questions with the respondent once the interview or questionnaire has been completed.

Even in well-planned studies there will be individuals who will forget to post back questionnaires, refuse to answer questions, or be unwilling to allow measurements on themselves to be taken. In a study mainly dependent on information obtained through the post, those who do not respond within a reasonable period of time may require

Key Message 2.4: Data Collection

It should not be assumed that the measurements made are exact. A measurement made on a particular individual could vary between observers or even with the same observer if the same measurement (on an x-ray, for example) is repeated.

postal reminders and possibly additional telephone calls. Note, however, that if it is clear that a patient is unhappy to be involved in the study, his or her decision should be respected (see Chapter 6).

Larger-scale studies involving research networks should include regular meetings of the staff involved in the study to consider progress and attempt to address possibly unforeseen problems as they arise. The involvement of patient representatives in such meetings can highlight difficulties from a layperson's point of view that might be overlooked by staff with dental training.

Data Entry

Once the study has been initiated, suitable databases should be set in place. These should be straightforward for use by data-entry staff and those subsequently involved in data analysis. Data-entry staff should be experienced with the chosen database and method of entry.

Data can be numerical (e.g., number of teeth, age of patients) or string (responses are represented using letters, e.g., type of tooth extracted). Where a value is missing for a numerical variable, an obvious number that is not a realistic value for that variable is inserted (e.g., 99 for number of missing teeth). Where a question is inapplicable (e.g., for men, number of teeth extracted since last pregnancy), a different implausible number (e.g., 88) is used. Most databases allow missing and inapplicable values to be defined as such. These are then dealt with in the analysis in an appropriate way; for example, values such as 99 might be excluded.

Automated data-entry methods such as optical mark recognition (OMR) are in common use. These involve tailor-made questionnaire forms on which the responses are entered into rows of printed squares one character per square. The completed forms are scanned in order to transfer the information to the database. If the characters are entered carefully, this technique has higher speed and accuracy than manual data entry.

For manual data entry, information from questionnaires or notes from interviews are normally entered into databases by clerical staff. Information is typed in quickly and errors are easily made. Confusion between letters and numbers (e.g., O and 0, I and 1) is often considered too obvious to mention to clerical staff, yet such errors can create havoc if not corrected before the data analysis commences. An incorrect key, close to the one intended could be hit or the correct key could be hit twice by mistake. Dates of birth, consultations, and death can become misaligned, as superficially they are similar in appearance.

The double-entry method is effective in minimizing manual

data-entry discrepancies. The data are entered twice and any differences checked; it is unlikely that the same unintentional error will be made on both occasions. Double-entry is time-consuming and the accuracy of numerical data can be assessed by range checks; values lying outside a range of plausible values (e.g., 44 children in a family) are queried. These checks are not infallible as errors falling within the range can go undetected. String data can be assessed by logical checks, in which improbable entries are queried.

Perform Data Analysis

Suitable statistical techniques should be selected, taking into account the nature of the variables, such as qualitative or quantitative (Williams, Bower, and Newton 2004). The size of the sample to be analyzed is important, as some techniques only give results that can be relied upon with larger samples. If there is pairing between individuals in different groups, the techniques are different from those appropriate for totally independent groups. The assumptions made in the data analysis should be carefully examined. In particular, most straightforward statistical methods operate on the assumption that the observations are independent of each other. Careful thought should be given as to whether this is realistic for the data to be analyzed. Sometimes it is not possible to find statistical techniques that suit the data exactly and this might have an impact on the validity of the results. This is one area where discussion with a statistician could prove invaluable.

Draw Conclusions

Although statistically significant findings should be noted, findings of clinical importance should be the main concern. No study is perfect and the discussion of the study should include ways in which future investigations of a similar nature could be improved.

Dissemination of the Findings from the Project

Once the study has been completed and discussed by the project members the findings should be presented to other interested groups. Initially, this might involve presentations at postgraduate study events or conferences. Discussions with members of the audience can be useful in appraising the findings and in the writing-up of the project as an article intended for an academic journal. If research funding has been obtained, every effort should be made to produce at least one academic publication (see Chapter 18 for further details). Even if the project is conducted solely by one individual and is opportunistic, a successful publication can be of considerable encouragement.

FUNDING

A crucial consideration when designing a study is the source of funding, if any. This can be an important factor in the size of the study or whether it goes ahead at all. It might be possible to conduct a small-scale study of a dental practice on an opportunistic basis and with little expense. This type of research is only feasible if a limited amount of data is required and it can be collected from patients when they visit the practice for their appointments. Any initiative on a larger scale, however, will be expensive and require money specifically earmarked for the project.

Financially, the best way for a general dental practitioner to become involved is as a participant in a research network led or facilitated by a university department or health authority. These organizations may have funding available through research bodies such as the Wellcome Trust (United Kingdom), the National Institute for Health Research (United Kingdom) and the National Institutes of Health (United States), and resources set up for regional health research initiatives. Researchers should be aware that competition for this type of funding can be fierce. The involvement of experienced researchers with a record of successful projects and publications can greatly increase the likelihood of a proposal being viewed positively.

BIAS

In an investigation, bias is an aspect of the study that tends to produce results that depart systematically from the true values. For example, the true average age of the patients registered at a dental practice might be 40 years but the method for selecting patients for a study might recruit a disproportionate number of elderly people, making the average age of the sample much higher. The main sources of bias are as follows.

Sampling Bias

Unless all individuals in a population are equally likely to be selected for a sample, then those selected are likely to be unrepresentative. For instance, in a study of teeth-brushing habits, asking patients at dental appointments will produce a sample in which those who regularly have dental inspections are over-represented and those who never attend are excluded. The assessment of brushing is likely to be over-optimistic as those who attend regularly are more likely to brush their teeth regularly.

Volunteer Bias

If inclusion in a study is based on the interest of the patients, the sample will consist mainly of individuals who have an above-average interest in their dental health. This is a problem with studies in which questionnaires are placed for completion on a table in the dental practice waiting room. Those with little interest in their dental health are unlikely to complete a questionnaire.

Recall Bias

If patients are asked to recall events that have happened in the past, their memory is likely to be incomplete. Patients who have received painful dental treatment may be more likely to remember when they last visited the dentist compared to those who never need work to be carried out. For questions about events that have occurred, say, within the last year, the phenomenon of an event seeming to have taken place more recently than is the case ("telescoping") is a common problem.

Assessment Bias

This occurs if measurements systematically deviate from true values because of the way in which they are taken. For example, when a patient is weighed while wearing usual clothing, the clothes form a significant addition to body weight. Similarly, rounding the length of a consultation upward to the nearest five minutes will give an overestimate of the average consultation time at a dental practice.

Communication Bias

In many populations, some patients have only a limited understanding of the language used by the study group (e.g., English in the United Kingdom and most of North America). The exclusion of such patients is a serious source of sampling bias. It is therefore good practice for at least some of the interviewers to be familiar with the languages likely to be used within the population of interest. In addition, written information intended for patients should be translated into locally used languages. Not only are questions more likely to be understood in an interview but showing consideration for the patient's cultural background can increase goodwill and the likelihood of cooperation.

Allocation Bias

For studies in which patients are allocated to one of several groups at the start, it is important that the groups are initially as similar as possible. Otherwise, differences between groups at the outcome stage might be accounted for by differences at the start. Allocation bias occurs if the groups differ systematically when they are set up. For example, in a comparison of two types of local anesthetic, the dentist might decide not to allow patients with poor physical health to receive the less established anesthetic. Patients with good health will then be over-represented in the group receiving the newer anesthetic.

Response Bias

Individuals who agree to take part in a study are likely to differ on average from those who refuse to take part. For a postal questionnaire the percentage responding can be less than 50%, so it is impossible to draw conclusions about the whole of the population. Where possible, patients should be given postal and/or telephone reminders, but this should be done tactfully as it is always the patient's right to decline involvement.

Key Message 2.5: Non-responders

Basic information can sometimes be obtained on non-responders; for example, in a dental practice it may be possible to find out age, sex, and address. Non-responders might differ from responders on an important variable about which information cannot be obtained from general records.

PATIENT AND PUBLIC INVOLVEMENT

Patient and public involvement (PPI) in research enables individuals from the population under investigation along with other members of the public to contribute to the design and conduct of the study. Instead of simply being viewed as participants, those who become engaged in these activities provide input based on their own personal experiences and so develop a degree of ownership in the research. It is considered good practice to involve patients and other interested parties in this way, and funding bodies increasingly require evidence of patient and public involvement in applications for research support.

Involvement may include commenting on patient information leaflets, acting as project advisors, and being co-applicants in research projects. For example, in an investigation into the public's views on the quality of dental care, a PPI group assisted in the development of questions for the study questionnaire (Tickle et al. 2015). Some research groups have established an ongoing patient and public involvement group for the provision of input into new projects as they evolve.

TEST YOUR UNDERSTANDING

1 In a practice data set the following information is found in the records of a woman aged 35 years. What is the most likely interpretation of each value?
  Options:
  (a) Missing value indicator
  (b) Plausible value
  (c) String entry error
  (d) Out of range
    (i) Number of teeth extracted = 99
    (ii) Number of fillings = 6
    (iii) Type of tooth extracted = SOLAR
    (iv) Age at last visit in years = 344
    (v) Visits in the last year = 2
2 Explain why ethical approval is required before project grants are released by research-funding organizations.
3 List three ways in which bias may arise in a community study of dental needs. Select one and suggest how the bias could be reduced.
4 Describe how a patient and public involvement group might contribute to an investigation into dental care provision for older people.

CHAPTER 3

Types of Study in Dental Research

INTRODUCTION

An important reason for undertaking an investigation into an area of research of relevance to dentists is the estimation of the value of a particular feature of a population. A question of this nature might be: "What proportion of 12-year-old girls have evidence of dental caries?" Although it might seem straightforward to calculate a proportion from a sample of girls, what is more difficult is to provide a range of believable values for the true proportion in the whole population. Statistical methods are required in order to give an indication of the accuracy of an estimate.

For many studies the main task is a comparison of two or more groups. The research question might be: "With regard to teenagers, does fluoridation affect the DMFT score (sum of the numbers of decayed, missing, and filled teeth)?" A comparison of young people living in an area with a fluoridated public water supply with a group living in a non-fluoridated area is required. Statistical methods can be used to decide whether any differences between the two groups are due to a real effect or have occurred purely on the grounds of chance. As with estimation for a single group, statistical methods can be used to give a range of likely values for the real differences between the two groups. This approach can be extended to three or more independent groups of individuals and to groups that have strong links between each other, such as a sample of men and their partners.

EPIDEMIOLOGICAL STUDIES

The investigation of the distribution and determinants of health-related conditions in populations is known as **epidemiology**. Epidemiological studies fall into one of three main groups, as follows.

Descriptive Epidemiology

Studies in this category tend to be regular surveys used to investigate the distribution of diseases in communities, such as the surveys of adult dental health conducted every 10 years in the UK. The findings from these surveys can be used to identify trends in oral health in the UK population by age, gender, socioeconomic class, and geographical region.

> **Key Message 3.1: Descriptive Studies**
>
> These cannot be used to decide whether or not a particular variable causes or increases the chance of dental problems; that is, to establish causal factors.

Analytical Epidemiology

Here, risk or causal factors for patterns of disease are investigated through **observational studies**, in which the natural behavior of individuals is observed over a period of time. For instance, in a study of the relationship between smoking and oral health, those who already smoke would form the group of smokers under investigation and those who do not smoke would make up the group of non-smokers. Subsequent changes in dental health for these groups would then be recorded and comparisons made.

Investigations of this type are referred to as **cohort studies**. In such a study no intervention takes place; in this example, the organizers would not offer the participants information or other assistance with giving up smoking. Cohort studies in which the participants commence their follow-up after the start of the investigation are described as being prospective.

Example 3.1

A prospective cohort study investigated post-operative morbidity following chin graft surgery (Joshi 2004). Twenty-seven patients who had undergone such surgery were followed up at one week, one month, three months and one year after their operation. The main research issue was the level of sensory loss following the operation and whether this changed over time. At each follow-up visit, dental staff assessed any sensory loss that the patient might have developed using simple tests. In addition, patients were asked to describe any experiences of altered sensation around the chin. In the light of the study findings it was possible to describe typical sensory changes following chin graft surgery. This would not have been possible had the patients been assessed on only one occasion.

In some investigations, known as **retrospective** studies, the data are obtained from dental records or by asking the patient to recall events from memory. Although the accuracy of records might be questionable and personal memory fallible, events that have occurred in the past can be highly relevant to the current dental health and attitudes of individuals and should, where appropriate, be taken into account.

For retrospective cohort studies, participant follow-up commences and is completed before the start of the investigation. Information is collected from participant records made during the period of interest. Data on the relevant outcomes are obtained from the records corresponding to the time at which follow-up ends.

Example 3.2

In a retrospective cohort study of the residents of Kobe City, Japan, Tanaka et al. (2015) reported the possible impact of maternal smoking during pregnancy and exposure of four-month-old infants to tobacco smoke on the development of dental caries by age three years. The study information was obtained from municipal records. Data on smoking during pregnancy and exposure to second-hand smoke were reported by parents using standardized questionnaires. Details regarding the condition of the teeth were obtained from assessments made by qualified dentists using visual examination at 18 months and three years. The presence of caries was indicated by the observation of at least one decayed, missing or filled tooth. The risk of caries during early life was associated with exposure to smoking in the household.

An investigation in which data are collected on patients on just one occasion is known as a cross-sectional study. For example, a satisfaction questionnaire about dental services might be offered to individuals in an outpatient waiting-room at a dental hospital. Questionnaires could be distributed during a series of clinics to increase the number of participants. Care should be taken to ensure that no patient completes more than one questionnaire, otherwise responses from completed questionnaires will not be independent of each other.

Example 3.3
A study investigated a possible relationship between dental health status and depression in homeless people living in Scotland (Coles et al. 2011). For each participant, the degree of tooth decay was assessed by an oral examination. For the assessment of depression, participants completed the Centre for Epidemiological Studies Depression Scale. A positive relationship was found between level of dental decay and depression.

Retrospective data collection plays an important role in **case-control** studies. With these, patients suffering from a particular disease (cases) are compared with a similar group of people who have not contracted the disease (controls). Dental records and patient recollection can be used to search for possible differences in, say, dental treatment or life-style that might have influenced the chance of contracting the disease. For instance, long-term heavy smoking and alcohol consumption have been shown to be associated with an increased risk of oral cancer (Scully and Porter 2000). A review of the medical records of patients undergoing surgery for oral cancer and individuals undergoing a routine dental inspection is therefore likely to show a higher proportion of heavy smokers and drinkers in the records of the "surgery" group of patients.

Key Message 3.2: Case-control Studies

The groups selected should be as similar as possible in terms of age distribution, gender, and other relevant factors. This reduces the likelihood of any interesting findings being brushed aside as possibly being due to differences in the original groups.

Where similarity in the characteristics of the groups is the chief concern the study is described as **unmatched**. For some topics, similarity of the groups is considered insufficient so the study is designed with specific pairs of individuals, one in each group, being similar. If the number of potential controls is large relative to the number of cases, increasing the sample size each case can be linked to several similar controls (see Chapter 16). Studies using pair-wise links are described as **matched**.

TABLE 3.1 Matching cases and controls in a case-control study

Fillings		*No fillings*	
Age (years)	*Sex*	*Age (years)*	*Sex*
10	Male	10	Male
12	Female	12	Female
5	Female	5	Female
7	Male	7	Male

Matching is of particular concern in studies with children, whose teeth develop quickly, and that a patient aged eight years (say) might not be comparable to a child who is two or three years older. Hence, in a dental study of young people about the role of nut consumption in the requirement for fillings, a 10-year-old boy with fillings would ideally be matched with a 10-year-old boy who does not have fillings. Other pairs of similar individuals would be found. The prevalence of nut consumption in the two groups would then be compared (Table 3.1).

The variables used for matching should be chosen with care. Unless a huge pool of controls is available, perfect matching of cases to controls is often impossible to achieve for three or more matching variables. In studies of adults, matching on age is not usually exact but is carried out to within three, five or 10 years.

Example 3.4

A matched case-control study was conducted in Kuwait in order to investigate a possible link between the use of dental x-rays and thyroid cancer (Memon et al. 2010). The cases were drawn from the records of the Kuwait Cancer Registry and defined as patients with primary thyroid cancer who were currently alive, aged no more than 70 years and resident in Kuwait. One control participant was recruited for each case from individuals attending primary care clinics for minor complaints, those accompanying a patient, and those visiting the clinic for any other reason. Controls were individually matched to cases based on year of birth (within three years), gender, nationality, and district of residence. Hence, matching was performed with a single control on gender, age, nationality, and location of residence. Self-reported information was obtained from the cases and controls using a personal interviewer who recorded the responses in a structured questionnaire. Details regarding exposure to x-rays (if any) were obtained as part of the medical history. Socioeconomic background, family history, and dietary information were also obtained for each participant. Cases and controls were compared on, among other things, previous exposure to dental x-rays to see whether such exposure was more common in the thyroid cancer patient group.

Experimental Epidemiology

In this category of study, an intervention is given to one group of individuals with other group(s) receiving a different type of intervention or none at all. The individuals are then followed up in terms of the outcome(s) under investigation.

Example 3.5

In 1955, fluoridation was introduced to the public water supply on the island of Anglesey, Wales. However, the water remained non-fluoridated in the nearby mainland area around Bangor. In the subsequent years, the benefit of fluoridation was assessed by comparing the levels of caries in the two communities (Jackson, James, and Thomas 1985). Following the termination of fluoridation in 1991, research has continued with young children living in Anglesey into the possible detrimental effects of its removal (Thomas, Kassab, and Jones 1995).

For clinical studies that compare an established treatment (known as the control) with a new one, a common design is to allocate willing patients to one of the treatment groups in a random manner. Such studies, known as randomized controlled trials, will be considered in more detail in Chapter 5.

Example 3.6

Nelson et al. (2011) reported a randomized controlled design to compare the effect of text message reminders to that of voice message reminders in reducing non-attendance at a pediatric dentistry clinic. Caregiver/child dyads, consisting of the child patient and the accompanying adult caregiver, were randomly allocated to either the text message group or the voice message (control) group. Caregivers who received a message by voicemail were more likely to attend the clinic than those who received a reminder by text (although in both groups younger caregivers were less likely to attend).

The crossover trial is a modification of the randomized controlled design. In these, patients take one of the treatments for a certain period and then transfer to the other. The order of receipt of treatments is determined randomly for each patient. An advantage of this design is that patients act as their own control. There may be a "carryover" effect of the first treatment into the second period, however. Sometimes there is a "wash-out" (time) period between the two treatments in an attempt to reduce this effect.

Key Message 3.3: Crossover Trials

These are generally used for chronic conditions such as gingivitis, where neither death nor complete cure is likely.

Example 3.7

Matsui et al. (2014) investigated the effect of tongue cleaning on the level of tongue coating. The study involved treatment and control periods undertaken as separate phases. During the treatment period, the initial level of coating was scored using the Winkel tongue coating index (WTCI), after which participants cleaned their tongue mechanically using a disposable tongue cleaner. To assess short-term changes in tongue coating, the tongue was scored again using the WTCI on days 3 and 10. In the control period, the level of tongue coating was scored at the same time points but no tongue cleaning was undertaken. The 30 volunteers involved in the study were randomly allocated to receive either the treatment or the control period first, the two phases being separated by a wash-out period of three weeks.

TEST YOUR UNDERSTANDING

1 Select the most appropriate study design for investigating the topics given below.
Options:
(a) Case-control study
(b) Cohort study
(c) Cross-sectional study
(d) Crossover trial
  (i) Wisdom teeth removal in adults during their twenties and thirties.
  (ii) The proportion of adults in Glasgow registered with a dentist.
  (iii) The effectiveness of dental floss and dental tape in reducing the development of plaque.

(iv) The impact of smoking on the discoloration of teeth using patients arriving for their first appointment following registration at a practice.

2 Explain why in a case-control study it is generally not possible to match cases with controls on age, gender, socioeconomic group, ethnicity, and the dental practice where the patient is registered (all five variables at the same time).

3 Why might a cohort study be an unsuitable design for an undergraduate student project?

CHAPTER 4

Sampling

INTRODUCTION

When conducting a study, it is necessary to define the target population (all patients who may be eligible for the study). However, it is often not possible to observe the whole target population. A study population is then defined as a subset of the target population (e.g., patients with oral carcinoma presenting at a particular hospital within a specified period of time).

SAMPLE SURVEYS

Some medical data are routinely collected, such as numbers of births and deaths, and for these measures the behavior of the whole population is known to a fair degree of accuracy. However, when the data are not routinely collected, it is usually both difficult and costly to study the whole population, so members are selected to provide a sample. The sample needs to be chosen in such a way that it is representative of the population. The primary techniques are: face-to-face interview of participants (patients or dentists) at the dental practice/hospital, telephone interviews, and postal or Internet-based surveys. Depending on the nature of the topic, opportunistic face-to-face patient interviews can achieve close to 100% response (Porter 2006), postal surveys with reminders can attain 60% response (McKernan et al. 2015), whereas Internet-based surveys tend to have low response rates (De Gregorio et al. 2015), typically around 25%.

Methods of Sampling

Quota Sampling

This type of sample is often collected in a busy town center. Its advantages are that collection can be completed quickly and cheaply. Hence it is a common method of sampling for student projects. However, the sample is likely to be biased. For instance, if the sample is taken during working hours it may include an over-representation of individuals with time to spare. Note that data collection in shopping centers will likely require advance permission from management.

Self-selected Sampling

Volunteers come forward to enter the study (e.g., questionnaires may be left in a dental surgery waiting room for patients to complete). This method, too, is popular for student investigations, as it requires relatively little organization. This type of sampling will tend to attract people who are particularly concerned about their health, again causing bias. Individuals may leave the premises unintentionally taking their form with them and young children can cause a distraction as they leave the waiting room in a mess!

The above two methods of sampling can lead to considerable selection bias. Bias can be reduced by using a method that requires a sampling frame.

Key Message 4.1: Sampling Frame

A list of each member of the study population is obtained and members on the list are numbered sequentially. To create the sample, numbers are selected and the individuals on the list having these numbers are approached. The proportion of the population that is selected to create the sample is known as the sampling fraction.

A sampling frame is often used in conjunction with a method of sampling that involves random selection. The main methods of this type are as follows.

Simple Random Sampling

A set of random numbers is generated and the associated individuals are selected from the list. Each member of the study population (listed in the sampling frame) has the same chance of being selected and

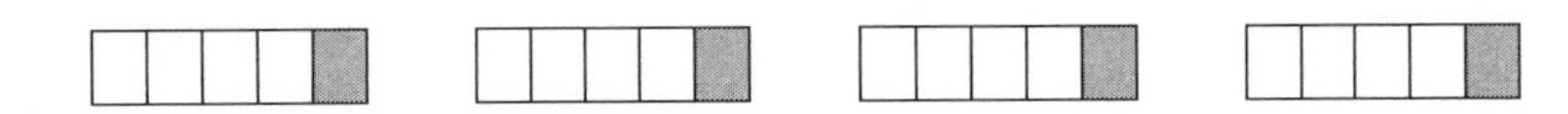

FIGURE 4.1 A biased systematic sample from a series of terraced houses. (Grey shading indicates selection.)

every sample of a particular size (e.g., size 20) has the same chance of being chosen.

Systematic Sampling

The sampling frame is divided into contiguous blocks of, perhaps, five, 10 or 20 patients. The initial individual selected is chosen from the first block at random. Subsequent individuals are then taken from the equivalent position in subsequent blocks. If, for instance, the blocks are of size 10, this amounts to selecting every 10th individual. If the size of the sampling frame is an exact multiple of the block size, each individual has the same chance of being chosen. However, unlike simple random sampling, all samples of the same size do not have an equal chance of being chosen; those containing adjacent members on the list will definitely not be selected.

Bias can enter the sampling in a subtle way. For instance, if this method is used with a list of appointments, the sample might include the first appointment of each day. These patients are more likely to have paid employment and schedule their dental appointment on their way to work. Individuals in paid employment might therefore be over-represented in the sample. As another example, if houses have been built in terraces of length five and every fifth house is selected for a survey, all of the homes in the sample could be an end-of-terrace (Figure 4.1). This is important if the type of house occupied influences the issue under investigation (e.g., spending on dental care).

Stratified Random Sample

The population is first divided into strata (population groups), based on a particular characteristic such as age or sex (two or more characteristics may be used in larger studies). A simple random sample is then selected from each stratum. It is not possible to draw a stratified random sample unless the sampling frame contains information on the chosen characteristics for each individual. This method is useful where some of the strata of interest represent only a small minority of the population (e.g. particular ethnic groups). Simple random sampling alone might fail to select any members of these strata. The key

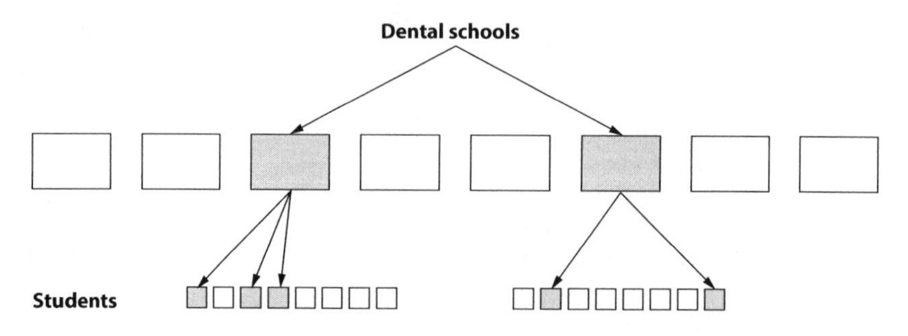

FIGURE 4.2 Selecting individuals using multistage sampling. (Grey shading indicates selection.)

is to take larger sampling fractions from the smaller strata in order to allow the sample groups to be of similar size.

Cluster Sampling

A list of all the individuals in the study population may not exist, but a list of larger units, such as households, may be available. A random selection of households (for instance) rather than individuals is taken. The people in these households form the sample. It should be remembered that individuals within households are often similar to each other in terms of diet and care of their teeth. Individual observations cannot therefore be regarded as independent; this complicates the appropriate method of analysis.

Multistage Random Sampling

Random sampling takes place at two or more levels. For instance, obtaining a random sample of all UK dental students would involve contacting all of the institutions concerned. Instead, one could draw a random sample of UK dental schools, contact only those schools, and take a random sample of students from within each chosen institution (Figure 4.2). This type of approach is frequently used with large study populations.

Is the Sample Representative?

Random sampling does not guarantee that every sample contains exactly the same proportion of people with a certain characteristic (it may be that in a small random sample of dental practice patients only females are selected). However, on average, random sampling will be representative. Using a large sample size reduces the chance of an atypical sample being obtained. It is therefore unfortunate that due to limitations of time and money, student projects often have to be based on simpler but more biased methods such as quota and self-selected sampling.

Key Message 4.2: Reporting Sampling Methods

A sample appearing to be unrepresentative could have arisen either by chance or by the use of non random sampling. The method of sampling should be fully described in the study report so that the reasons for any discrepancy in the sample can be explored.

TEST YOUR UNDERSTANDING

1 Explain, using an example from dentistry, what is meant by a simple random sample. Why is this type of sample not always representative of the population from which it is drawn?
2 Describe how in a dental practice a systematic sample could be drawn from the patients arriving for treatment. Give one advantage and one disadvantage in using this method of sampling rather than simple random selection.
3 In a study undertaken in a large town on attitudes to dental care, why will selection of names from the local telephone directory lead to sampling bias?

CHAPTER 5

Randomized Controlled Trials

INTRODUCTION

When a new treatment for a particular dental problem is discovered, it is necessary to compare the effects of the treatment with those of the treatment in current use, using patients who have that problem. In **clinical trials** the treatments are allocated to the patients. Since the effectiveness of a new treatment can only be assessed properly within the context of treatments currently available, patients are allocated to either a "new treatment" (intervention) group or a **control** group where the established treatment is given (if one exists). As an example, some dentists believe that young children may take in harmful levels of fluoride by swallowing their toothpaste and decide to investigate a low-fluoride variety. However, there might be unresolved concern that low-fluoride toothpaste is less effective in preventing tooth decay. It might then be appropriate to compare the effectiveness of a low-fluoride variety of children's toothpaste with a standard fluoride type in terms of change in primary teeth decay score dmft over a predetermined length of time. If the treatment proposed has no medically effective alternative, a **placebo** treatment, which has no biological

Key Message 5.1: Placebo Effect

It is well known that some patients improve when given a placebo. This is known as the placebo effect. It is a psychological response to the knowledge that treatment is being received. For the new treatment, an effect must be demonstrated over and above the placebo effect.

effect on the patient, can be used for the control group. This is acceptable from an ethical point of view if it is still undetermined that the new treatment has a clear advantage.

When new drugs, procedures or dental education programs are introduced, results obtained from a few patients may appear promising. A study must then be designed which compares two groups of patients, one receiving the old treatment and the other receiving the new treatment. The process of selecting suitable patients for the treatment and control groups is known as **allocation**. As will be seen later, many methods of allocation can lead to substantial differences between the groups before the experiment has even begun. This lays the study open to bias. A method of assigning patients in a random manner greatly reduces the chance of serious allocation bias.

ALLOCATION BY RANDOMIZATION

In the simplest form of random allocation, in a comparison of two groups, the treatment decision for each patient is made on what amounts to the toss of a coin (head being "assign to new treatment," tail being "assign to control group"), although most studies now use computer-generated random numbers. The treatment assignments are then placed individually in sealed envelopes in the generated order.

As each patient arrives, the clinician first decides whether the patient should be enrolled on the study (specific exclusion criteria should have been set). Suitable patients are given information about the study and asked to give informed consent if they are happy to participate (see Chapter 6). If the patient's decision is positive, the next envelope in the series is opened and the treatment indicated is allocated to that patient. If it is intended that group sizes should be substantially different, **unequal randomization** may be used, where the probability of receiving the new treatment is different from 0.5.

Key Message 5.2: Allocation Bias Due to the Dentist

Randomization removes the pitfall of the dentist having to make a subjective professional judgment about the trial group that is most suitable for the patient.

A 50:50 randomization may not produce two groups of similar size, especially in small studies. One solution to this problem is to use

TABLE 5.1 Randomized blocks of size six with three decisions of each type

(1) AAABBB	(2) AABABB	(3) AABBAB	(4) AABBBA	(5) ABAABB
(6) ABBBAA	(7) ABABBA	(8) ABBAAB	(9) ABABAB	(10) ABBABA
(11) BBBAAA	(12) BBABAA	(13) BBAABA	(14) BBAAAB	(15) BABBAA
(16) BAAABB	(17) BABAAB	(18) BAABBA	(19) BABABA	(20) BAABAB

randomized blocks. For example, treatment decisions could be taken in blocks of six. Within each block there are three allocations of each type but the six decisions are in a random order. There are 20 possible blocks (Table 5.1).

One of the 20 blocks is chosen at random (see Chapter 4), and the allocations are made in the order given by the block. For instance, the selection of Block 7 would give the allocations: Group A, Group B, Group A, Group B, Group B, Group A. Once the first six individuals have been allocated, a further block is selected at random and the process is repeated until all the study participants have been allocated. In the study as a whole, the group sizes will be equal if the number of patients is a multiple of six and approximately equal otherwise. Traditionally, blocks of eight treatment decisions have been used; this gives 70 rather than 20 different possible blocks.

Key Message 5.3: Imbalance

Randomization does not guarantee that the patients in the two groups will be equal in every respect (e.g., the same proportions of females), but in trials with large numbers of patients a large imbalance is unlikely to occur.

If a factor is known to affect either severity of disease or recovery from it (possibly age, sex), it is advisable to divide the subjects into strata (subgroups) on the basis of that factor. Random allocation is then performed separately for each of the subgroups. In this way, the comparison of treatments can be kept unbiased by ensuring that, for example, males and females are evenly distributed between the treatments. Except in very large studies, stratification is only feasible for one or two factors and this still does not ensure comparability of treatment groups for other factors that have not been taken into account.

ALTERNATIVES TO RANDOM ALLOCATION

Sometimes it is more convenient to use methods that do not depend on randomization. The main alternatives include historical and non-randomized controls.

Historical Controls

In this situation, the results for current patients on the new treatment are compared with results from previous patients on an old treatment or before any treatment was available. In fact, any differences could be due to changes over time unrelated to the treatments.

For example, suppose that a long-established dental practice has for the last five years distributed to its patients a leaflet about the need for the regular brushing of teeth. It might be hoped that in the light of the advice given the need for dental treatment would decrease. However, should the investigators attempt to demonstrate the effect of the leaflet by comparing treatment records with data recorded on patients who attended when the practice first opened, any apparent decrease might be due to a long-term decline in the use of sugar, reducing the severity of dental caries in the patient population irrespective of the leaflet. The types of patient treated at the practice may also have changed over time; for example, with a greater focus on private treatment.

It is important to note that the criteria for assessing outcome may change. For instance, the extraction of a tooth might once have been seen as routine whereas now it may be regarded as a particularly unsatisfactory outcome.

Non Randomized Controls

The controls could be selected as part of the main study but in a non random manner. A method convenient to the dentist is judgment assignment. Here the dentist decides which treatment is best for individual patients. This method is subjective and open to bias on the part of the dentist.

Another possible method is to allocate treatment according to hospital or dental practice; for example, patients at one hospital have the new treatment whereas patients at another would receive the old treatment. Bias can arise due to other differences in patient care between the hospitals. Methods of patient selection and assessment might also vary between institutions.

A method of allocation straightforward for clerical staff to implement is to assign patients to one of two treatments alternately in order of entry to the study. Alternatively, patients might be assigned to a group according to whether their date of birth is odd or even. In these situations, the dentist will be informed of the treatment allocated to each patient in advance and may decide not to enroll patients thought to be unsuitable for the treatment. This will almost certainly lead to allocation bias in the selection of patients for the treatment groups.

TREATMENT ADMINISTRATION

The dosage and frequency of treatments should be agreed upon by the clinical staff involved before the commencement of the study, taking into account current information about the effects of these treatments on the human body. The nature, severity, and likelihood of possible side effects should be assessed and a procedure for withdrawing patients who experience them should be incorporated into the study design. Allowance should also be made in the design for patients to exercise their right to withdraw from the study themselves.

Blinding

Investigators with clinical training will have detailed knowledge of the established treatment and informed opinions as to the possible impacts of the new treatment. Others involved are likely to have some knowledge about the treatments obtained from scientific sources, the media, or family and friends. It is therefore important that the information recorded in the study is not biased by any prior knowledge or preconceived ideas as to the effects of the treatments. "Blinding" (sometimes known as masking), which has the purpose of concealing information about the treatment being received by particular patients, should be incorporated into the study design where possible.

Blinding has several aspects and can involve the patients, clinicians, and outcome assessors, as well as data analysts. In study descriptions, the term single blinding usually indicates that the patients are unaware of their treatment group. A study in which both patients and clinicians/outcome assessors are unaware of individual allocations is described as being double blind. If the patients, clinicians/outcome assessors, and data analysts are all unaware of individual patient allocations, the study is generally referred to as triple blind. Studies that involve no blinding are called open or open-label investigations. The above terms are not used consistently in the scientific literature, and it is therefore advisable when reading a report to check the study design carefully as to the description of any blinding involved.

Investigations involving surgery are almost always impossible to conduct in a manner that incorporates blinding. For blinding to be a practical option, the treatments (often forms of oral medication) must be the same in appearance and manner of administration. For instance, if two tablets are being compared, they should be of the same shape, size, color, and taste. It can be difficult to maintain study blindness even where investigators take reasonable precautions to prevent disclosure. Other necessary aspects of patient care may make it impossible to conceal the treatment group of individual patients. In any reports, potential or actual weaknesses in the blinding process should be stated. Patient withdrawal due to side effects or for other reasons should also be disclosed.

Key Message 5.4: Blinding

Knowledge of the treatment received may affect a patient's responses to it, or the clinician's judgment of such responses. Where measures are subjective (e.g., level of pain, side effects) it is particularly important that, if possible, the trial incorporates blinding.

ANALYSIS

The analysis of the results should be performed on an **intention to treat** basis. If patients are randomly allocated to one of two treatment groups, some of them may decide afterwards to discontinue or change their treatment. However, the groups are still compared as they were originally chosen. This gives a realistic indication of the probable effect of the new treatment if adopted in routine practice.

Key Message 5.5: Intention to Treat Analysis

To analyze the patients by their actual treatment at the end of the study would introduce bias, as those who are not happy to continue with their original treatment are likely to have characteristics different from those of the other patients.

The analysis of the results is a comparison of the variable of interest (outcome variable) between the treatment groups. The type of analysis will depend upon the nature of the outcome variable.

Two treatment groups may show an apparent difference due to:

- A difference between the groups other than the difference in treatments, e.g., more females in the new treatment group (stratification and randomization may help here).
- Bias by the dentist or patient in the assessment of the outcome variable (blindness addresses this).
- Sampling (chance) variation.
- A true difference in the effects of the treatments.

Key Message 5.6: The Study Design Should Be Checked Carefully

Statistical analysis is used to distinguish between chance variation and true differences. However, statistics can do little to allow for bias that has entered into the results owing to poor study design.

Before generalizing results, it is necessary to consider the population from which the patients in the study were selected. Studies on dental outpatients may not yield results that can be generalized to the community. Results from one hospital cannot necessarily be generalized to other hospitals, where, for instance, other aspects of treatment may differ. Recently obtained results may not be applicable to groups of patients in the future.

CLUSTER RANDOMIZED TRIALS

For some research studies it may be appropriate to use randomization but impractical to allocate patients to the intervention or control group on an individual basis. This may be the case if, for example, the intervention is a health promotion initiative such as the provision of a leaflet containing advice on smoking cessation. Instead of allocating individual patients at random to either receive the leaflet (intervention group) or not (control group) it would be easier to randomize dental practices. Practices involved in the intervention would be provided with leaflets to give to all relevant patients, whereas the control practices would not be sent copies of the leaflet and patients would receive their usual care only.

The data collected from a cluster randomized trial can be analyzed in more sophisticated and realistic ways. Trials in which individuals are randomized generally involve statistical methods that rely on the assumption of independence between the observations from different participants. In reality this is unlikely to be the case, as individuals in the intervention and control groups registered with the same practice may be acquainted with each other and discuss the investigation. In addition, for a specific practice the characteristics of the dental staff and the practice management may attract particular types of patient. One with a waiting area that is designed with children in mind is likely to appeal to families, whereas a practice that accepts only private patients may be the preference of the more affluent. Patients within a dental practice may therefore be more similar than dental patients taken as a whole. Cluster randomized trials are able to take any association between individual responses and similarities between patients within clusters into account through the use of intraclass correlation, a concept that will be explained in Chapter 14.

In terms of study design and conduct, the issues that need to be addressed for good research practice in cluster randomized trials are similar to those involved in investigations that use individual randomization. Blinding should be incorporated wherever possible in order to reduce bias and the analyses should be performed on an intention to treat basis.

Withdrawal from the study requires careful consideration where clusters are involved as not only can individual patients withdraw/be withdrawn but a complete cluster (e.g., one of the participating dental practices) can be lost if the staff concerned have a change of mind. A design having a large number of smaller clusters is often preferred to one with a small number of larger clusters, as the loss of a single cluster is then less critical.

TEST YOUR UNDERSTANDING

Case Study: A Better Mouth Rinse?

Mary Williams is a single-handed dental practitioner who has a busy first-floor high-street practice close to central Birmingham, England. Hita, a dental nurse, and Joan, the receptionist, assist her. Mary's hours are 9 am to 1 pm, 1.30 pm to 5 pm. Patients are booked in 10-minute slots. Social deprivation is high in the immediate area. The percentage of the local population claiming disability allowance is above average compared with the United Kingdom as a whole. Around a third of the local population is Black Caribbean, although over 90% of Mary's patients, some of whom live in the more affluent suburbs, would describe themselves as white. Most of her work is done under the British National Health Service (NHS), although Mary has a few private patients. She has a special interest in anxiety-reduction techniques, and plays recorded classical music during treatment unless the patient requests otherwise. She has several soft toys of popular TV cartoon characters in the treatment room.

For several years, Mary has been using Xellent as the mouth rinse offered to patients immediately following treatment. Regulars are familiar with the pink solution. Recently she has heard that an alternative mouth rinse, Ynot, might leave patients with a better sense of well-being. She decides to investigate whether or not Ynot is indeed superior by providing some of her patients with Xellent and others with Ynot, and asking them to complete a patient satisfaction questionnaire following treatment (this uses the scale: very satisfied/satisfied/indifferent/dissatisfied/very dissatisfied). To ensure that each individual contributes just once to the study, patients on a series of treatment visits will be asked to participate only on their first visit following the start of the study.

Joan is to explain the study to each patient on arrival and discreetly indicate to Hita the solution that has been allocated to the patient. She will also have to give a copy of the questionnaire to each patient following treatment and collect the completed forms. Hita will fill identical glasses with the allocated mouth rinse solution.

Joan has made it clear that she will only tolerate the potential upheaval caused by the proposed trial for a maximum of two weeks; otherwise she will give her notice. Hita is happy to be involved but she will be leaving the practice in three months' time to work in the US. It is unlikely that an immediate replacement will be found for Hita.

Peter, a statistician friend, has informed Mary that at least 100 patients will be needed in each of the Xellent and Ynot groups in order to detect any important difference between the two solutions.

1 Jon, Mary's former dental public health tutor, works in a large private dental practice located in an affluent area on the edge of Birmingham. Five years ago he conducted a study using the same patient satisfaction questionnaire. The patients involved used Xellent following treatment. Should she restrict her study to Ynot, comparing her findings with those of her tutor? She might not then need as many patients.
2 Mary thinks that Joan might regard the study as less of an imposition if every sixth patient is entered into the study. Should this suggestion be made to Joan?
3 When Mary discusses her project with Jon, he suggests a crossover design in which each patient uses the alternative solution at his or her following visit. Is this good advice?

4 Reflecting on Jon's advice, Mary wonders whether matching similar patients might be worth considering. Would matching be helpful here?
5 At present Ynot solution has a rather striking orange color, but the manufacturers have stated that in two months' time it will be available in the more traditional pink. Should Mary wait until supplies of the pink Ynot solution can be obtained?
6 Mary intends to allocate patients to either Xellent or Ynot on the toss of a coin, the sequence being determined in advance. Should she do this?
7 Hita suggests that patients should not be told about the study in advance but be handed the questionnaire following treatment. Is this good practice?
8 Initially it was thought that patients should complete the questionnaire before leaving the premises. It could be reasoned, however, that patients might not feel well enough to complete the questionnaire immediately after treatment. Patients could instead be given the questionnaire to complete at home along with a stamped envelope for posting it back. Would this be better?
9 Joan gradually becomes more enthusiastic but she does think that children involved may pose particular problems for the study. Should this be a concern?
10 Mary has doubts as to whether the study will fully reflect the population of patients on her list. Are these justified?
11 Peter believes that this study is likely to be unrepresentative of the local community in which Mary's practice is located. Do you think that he is correct?
12 The study shows that 65% of patients using Xellent and 85% of patients using Ynot were either very satisfied or satisfied with their treatment. Should Mary change to using Ynot?

CHAPTER 6

Ethical Considerations

INTRODUCTION

Ethical issues are important in both the practice of dentistry and the conduct of dental research studies. This chapter gives an outline of the basic concepts and illustrates some common ground with statistics. For an in-depth study of ethics, Herring (2014) explores medical ethics from a European perspective, whereas Ozar and Sokol (2002) focus on dental ethics from an American angle. For coverage of dental law and how it relates to ethics see Lambden (2002).

PATIENT CONSENT

It is generally considered to be good practice to obtain the patient's consent before the commencement of any dental examination or treatment. It could be reasoned that consent to a dental examination has already been given if the patient has made an appointment to see the dentist. To assume that this implied/passive consent carries through to the treatment stage is unwise; this could potentially lead to a legal challenge by the patient, particularly if the treatment is unsuccessful. Positive informed consent, in which the patient makes a definite decision to receive the treatment, should be obtained where possible. If there are significant implications to the patient in terms of further visits, financial cost or pain, this consent should be written rather than verbal so that a record is kept.

If the patient is not an adult who is capable of making an informed choice, deciding on whether or not to proceed with treatment may be challenging (Leathard and McLaren 2007). For children and young people, the assent of a parent or other appropriate adult should be sought before the treatment takes place; the young person should also be willing. A similar situation occurs for those with a learning disability or an older person who is no longer competent to make a reasoned decision. In an emergency "life or death" situation in which a patient is unconscious, the assent of a relative should be sought. If no suitable individual is available to give assent, procedures may need to be performed without the patient's consent in the patient's best interests, although in dentistry such events are rare.

GENERAL PRINCIPLES

Ethical considerations are important both in general dental care and in the planning and conduct of investigations. The main ethical principles are **respect for autonomy** or self-rule, **non-maleficence**, **beneficence** and **justice** or fairness. In addition, the concept of **scope** is sometimes included. Since these concepts are frequently referred to in the discussion of research ethics, they will be briefly outlined below.

Respect for Autonomy

Autonomy is the ability of an individual to think, decide, and act independently. In the context of dental care, the dentist should avoid being paternalistic (i.e., having the attitude "the dentist knows best") but rather discuss intended procedures with the patient prior to the commencement of treatment. This ideal is not always possible, as many patients are happy for the dentist to take total responsibility for each aspect of their care. If this has been made clear by the patient following an opportunity for discussion, autonomy will not be compromised.

An important aspect of respect for autonomy is that of confidentiality. Details of patient care should only be made available to those who need them, such as other members of the health-care team. Sensitive information given by the patient in confidence should only be divulged in exceptional circumstances. In particular, dentists should not inform the patient's relatives of the diagnosis of a serious problem (e.g., oral cancer) without the patient's consent.

Non-maleficence

This principle is encapsulated in the medical maxim "above all, do no harm." In as far as is possible, the dentist should seek to avoid harm, for instance, in the pain experienced by patients. Sometimes harm has to be caused in order to achieve subsequent benefits, such as in the surgical removal of a tumor from the mouth. In fact, this may be the most appropriate course of action as the side effects of the alternatives, radiotherapy or chemotherapy, can be worse than the effects of the disease. Before a procedure is selected a harm/benefit analysis should be carried out jointly between the dentist and the patient. This is particularly important for radical procedures such as surgery. The patient should then give informed consent before treatment commences.

Beneficence

Dentists are morally obliged to contribute to the health and welfare of their patients. It should be noted that in order to respect patient autonomy, a beneficial treatment should not be given against the wishes of the patient.

Justice

The resources available to the individual dentist, or indeed society, are limited. In the development of dental services an important consideration is distributive justice. How can limited resources be distributed in a way that is "fair"? Various models for resource distribution have been proposed, including: (1) equal resources for all; (2) equal access to needed care; (3) distribution in favor of those who contribute the most (e.g., financially or intellectually); (4) an unrestricted free market in which the buyer and seller determine the price of treatment.

Scope

The concept of scope relates to the extent to which the dentist has a duty of care. For some dentists, a moral obligation to provide good care applies only to the patients in their practice, along with a few specific emergency situations. Others are prepared to spend some of their professional time caring for those who are least able to help themselves, such as the homeless, with limited prospects of reward.

RESEARCH ETHICS

Most dental research proposals need to be assessed by ethical committees. The ethical aspects of the proposed work require justification before approval is given, and evidence of prior consultation with a statistician regarding the design and analysis is often necessary.

In dental research investigations, each potential participant should give informed consent. To facilitate this, they should each receive a written information sheet that outlines the main points about the study. Ideally, complete information about the possible efficacy and side effects of the treatments involved in the study should be given to the patient. In practice, not all patients will understand or even wish to receive additional information beyond that contained in the information sheet, particularly in a sophisticated trial. In such a situation, the patient should be given a choice regarding the amount of information received.

In a randomized controlled trial patients need to be clear about the method of treatment allocation. Referring to it in terms of the toss of a coin might be helpful. It has been suggested that in a randomized comparison of two treatments, patients who do not wish to be randomized to a particular treatment should instead be allowed to choose their preferred treatment. Doing this would produce three groups: The patients who request Treatment A; the patients who request Treatment B; and those who are randomized.

The autonomy of the patient should be respected and the patient should only make a decision on whether to enter the trial following careful consideration of the information provided. This is particularly important with diagnostic tests for potentially devastating diseases such as oral cancer (see Chapter 8). It should be made clear to patients that they can leave the trial at any time without necessarily giving a reason and that their usual treatment will be unaffected. Some studies attempt to encourage participation with small financial incentives. For instance, in a school-based study of tooth decay in rural adolescents in Washington State, US, pupils received $10 on completion of the study questionnaire (Skaret et al. 2004).

Once a trial has been completed, patients who feel that they have received an effective treatment for their health problem may wish to continue with it. Financial constraints and/or the concerns of the patient's usual dentist or general practitioner may prevent long-term use of the treatment; this should be discussed in advance as part of the patient information.

It is ethically unacceptable to study certain issues by allocating individuals to one of the possible groups at random. For example, in a study of the effects of smoking on health, one could not instruct individuals to smoke or to abstain from smoking as this disregards the autonomy of the study participants. In such a situation, the individual's choice of whether to smoke cigarettes or not must be respected, and an alternative type of study which makes this possible must be chosen.

In other situations, ethical issues are less clear and in practice until recently these have often been ignored. At the early stages of development, a new treatment for an illness may be associated with harmful side effects and may clash with the principle of non-maleficence. When the benefits of a new treatment are fairly clear, many dentists reason from the principle of beneficence that it is wrong to deny patients care by giving them the previously standard treatment. If early results from a trial indicate that one of the treatments is clearly superior, it is unethical to allow the trial to continue. It is even worse to conduct a comparison of two treatments when it is fairly certain at the start that one of them is better. All new studies should be based on information gleaned from a comprehensive search of findings from related work by using, for instance, MEDLINE (see Chapter 17). It is unethical to conduct research "in the dark," as it is probable that time and money will not be used to best effect.

Ethical issues often raise questions to which there is no obviously correct answer. For example, suppose that there were high hopes that a new drug might greatly relieve suffering in oral surgery and only enough doses were available to treat a few patients. The principles of beneficence and justice may suggest that the patients to receive the drug should be those who require the most extensive surgery. In a situation like this, the drug may reduce the suffering of those in greatest need. Because such patients are likely to experience more severe symptoms than those with a less serious condition who are not given the drug, this strategy does not seem unreasonable. There would, however, be conflict in terms of a "fair" evaluation of the merits of the drug that might have been obtained through a randomized trial.

Key Message 6.1: Confidentiality of Data

Patient records in dental practices and information collected in research studies should be kept confidential; this is a legal requirement in most countries. For instance, in the United Kingdom computer records should adhere to the principles laid down in the Data Protection Act, 1998. Data used for statistical purposes should not contain the names and addresses of the individuals concerned.

Diagnostic Screening

Difficult ethical dilemmas can arise from diagnostic screening. Few tests are perfect and individuals undergoing a screening test should be made aware that a positive result does not automatically mean that they have the disease any more than a negative result necessarily rules out the possibility of having the disease. In particular, those with a negative result may develop the disease in the future. Patients entering screening studies such as the one for oral cancer discussed in Chapter 8 need to be made aware that a definite diagnosis could affect future proposals for life insurance, consideration for a mortgage, and the like, as part of the patient information given when consent is requested (see Example 8.1, p. 64).

Example 6.1

A study conducted in the United Kingdom investigated the satisfaction and understanding of the consent process of patients attending a primary care dental practice (Hajivassiliou and Hajivassiliou 2015). Adult patients completed a structured questionnaire with a space for written comments underneath the closed (tick-box) questions. Of the 52 patients involved, there was 100% satisfaction with all aspects of the consent process apart from the explanation of complications, regarding which 11% were dissatisfied. However, their level of understanding regarding patient consent gave some cause for concern. Although 96% correctly understood that the signed consent form gives permission to the dentist to perform the procedure and 84% rightly believed that consent confirms that sufficient information has been given to the patient prior to their treatment decision, 44% were incorrect in thinking that signed consent is a legal necessity. In addition, 60% wrongly assumed that consent is obtained as a means of protecting doctors, dentists, and hospitals.

Sample Size

Small studies often fail to yield useful findings and are thus a poor use of resources. A sufficiently large number should be involved in order to have a reasonable chance of finding whether the expected difference between the two groups really exists. On the other hand, recruiting more participants than needed can waste resources. In medical research, in either situation more patients than necessary are at risk of receiving an inferior treatment. A sample-size calculation (see Chapter 16) should be performed at the design stage to estimate an appropriate sample size. Careful planning should consider the composition of the sample with respect to age, sex, ethnic group, and so on, as this will enable problems under investigation to be answered more effectively. The intended method of statistical analysis also influences the sample-size requirement.

TEST YOUR UNDERSTANDING

1 Select the most appropriate description of the consent obtained in the situations below.

Options:

(a) Positive consent

(b) Passive consent

(c) No consent

(i) As part of a research project, children receive a short dental examination during school hours. Parents are asked to provide a note to the class teacher if they do not wish their child to be involved in the study.

(ii) The dentist asks patients at a dental practice whether they are happy with their proposed treatment plan before work commences.

(iii) Without previously checking with the patient, a dentist proceeds with fillings as soon as a dental examination has been performed.

2 Explain why neglecting to estimate the sample size required for a proposed study can be considered unethical. Give one way in which the researcher may obtain information that will assist in the sample-size calculation.

3 Is it ethical to collect information from individuals on variables that are unlikely to be analyzed in a study?

CHAPTER 7

The Normal Distribution

INTRODUCTION

Many variables found in dental data, such as salivary flow rate, sugar consumption per week, and exact age, are continuous. Sample data on a continuous variable can be illustrated as a histogram (see Appendix, p. 159). These histograms rarely take a perfectly smooth shape, but they can sometimes be approximated by simple curves. For instance, adult central incisor width has been shown to be roughly symmetrical with a concentration of cases between 7 mm and 8 mm (Chu 2007). In order to treat observations as independent we assume that just one central incisor (upper left, say) is measured per individual. The continuous, symmetric, bell-shaped **Normal distribution**, shown below, might then form a good approximation to such a sample distribution (Figure 7.1).

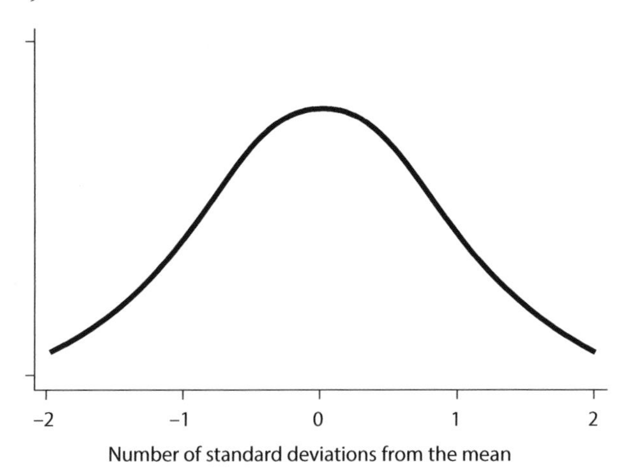

FIGURE 7.1 The Normal distribution.

APPLYING THE NORMAL DISTRIBUTION TO DATA

The Normal distribution is defined by its mean and standard deviation (the mean of a set of values is a type of average; the standard deviation measures the variation of these values around the mean – see Appendix for details, pp. 159–160).

The areas of the curve most distant from the mean are known as the tails of the distribution. With a small sample of perhaps 10 or 20 teeth the histogram of central incisor width would be very jagged and it would be difficult to tell whether this approximation is appropriate. As a sample is increased in size, to perhaps 500 or 1000 teeth, the histogram becomes much smoother and any possible underlying shape becomes more apparent.

Why is it useful to be able to approximate a sample histogram in this way? Chapter 1 introduced the concept of deducing characteristics of a population from a sample drawn from that population. A simple underlying curve might make a reasonable approximation for the population distribution. If this is the case, it is possible to estimate the proportion of the distribution exceeding a particular value. Although perhaps not immediately obvious, this forms the basis of many of the methods used to make inferences about a population. This will be explored in detail from Chapter 9 onward.

From Figure 7.1 it can be seen that a substantial part of the distribution is within one standard deviation of the mean and most of the distribution is within two standard deviations. Since the Normal distribution has an underlying mathematical formula (although we do not have to be concerned about these details) "substantial" and "most" have particular values (68% and 95%, respectively). By knowing the mean and standard deviation of a Normal distribution, it is possible to say whether a particular value from that distribution is around the average, extremely high, and so on. This is useful in assessing how an individual's observation compares to those of others from that population.

Key Message 7.1: Variation Within a Normal Distribution

About two-thirds (68%) of the population lies within one standard deviation of the mean and 95% of the population lies within two standard deviations of the mean.

Example 7.1

A water company is responsible for providing a public supply, fluoridated at a level of 1 part per million (ppm). Although the city authority accepts that fluctuations in this level might occur, the level is required to be above 0.9 ppm at all times. The actual level assessed on different occasions usually varies between 0.8 ppm and 1.2 ppm. Around how much of the time is the company failing in its obligation?

It is not possible to say precisely, but if "usually" is taken as around 95% of the time and the underlying distribution is assumed to be Normal, then from the properties of such a distribution, the value 0.8 is two standard deviations below the mean of 1 ppm. Hence the standard deviation is 0.1. So, the limit set by the city authority (0.9) is one standard deviation below the mean (Figure 7.2).

Two-thirds of a Normal distribution lies within one standard deviation of the mean. With the distribution being symmetrical, the remaining third will be equally divided between the left and right tails. Hence, around one-sixth of the distribution has a lower value than one standard deviation below the mean. The city authority's limit is not met for around one-sixth of the time. (NB: If the more precise figure of 68% is used instead the answer is almost the same, at 16%.)

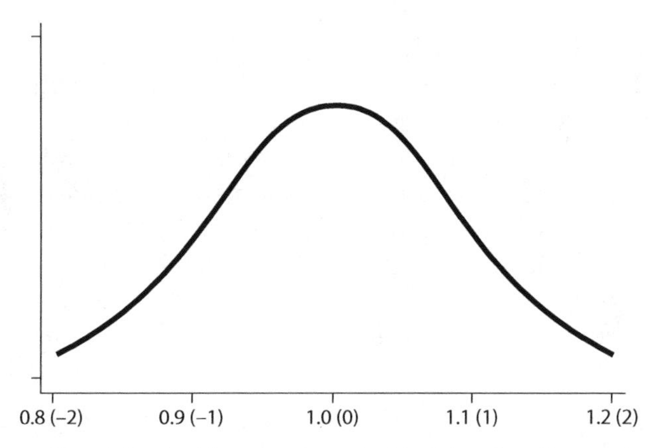

FIGURE 7.2 Distribution of fluoride measurements (ppm).

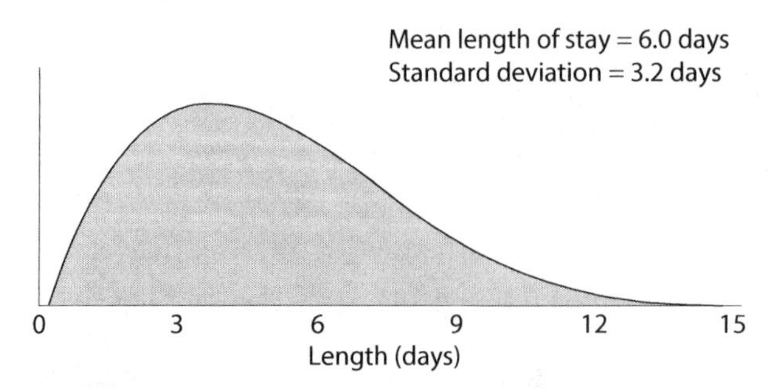

FIGURE 7.3 Distribution of length of hospital stay.

Deducing Non-Normality

Many distributions are not symmetrical let alone Normally distributed. It is important then not to apply the reasoning used in Example 7.1 as the answers obtained could be highly misleading. It is sometimes possible to show that a distribution is non-Normal from the values of the mean and standard deviation alone. We have seen that for a Normal distribution, some of the values will be lower than two standard deviations below the mean. If the mean minus twice the standard deviation is negative, and the data must be positive (e.g., lengths of inpatient admissions in days), there is a contradiction. In order to accommodate the lower limit of zero the data must be positively skewed (see Appendix, p. 160). The relatively large value for the standard deviation compared to the mean is due to the very large values in the positive tail (Figure 7.3).

TEST YOUR UNDERSTANDING

1 Give three reasons why the distribution of observations from a sample will not have an exact Normal distribution.
2 A dentist leaves work each day between 5.30 pm and 6 pm such that any departure time within this interval is equally likely. She notes down these times over a three-month period. Is the Normal distribution likely to provide a good model for the data collected? Justify your answer.
3 Why is it that in a population of adults a distribution of the number of teeth remaining with a mean of 30 and a standard deviation of 4 cannot be Normal?

CHAPTER 8

Diagnostic Tests

INTRODUCTION

A common problem in dentistry is the need to distinguish between those individuals who suffer from a specific condition and those who do not. It may be that the procedure required in order to be sure about the oral health of a patient needs the expertise of a dental specialist. In such a situation there is often a simple, less expensive procedure that a general dental practitioner can perform in order to obtain a good (though not perfect) idea about the likelihood of the patient having this dental health problem. For instance, in checking for the presence or absence of oral cancer, a specialist in oral surgery should be able to give a definitive answer, but this would be quite costly in terms of hospital resources and patient time. A simple check-up by a general dental practitioner might reveal unusual ulcers, for instance, justifying a referral of the patient to a dental hospital for further investigations. Patients with no such signs would be able to continue receiving just their routine dental care.

Of course, sometimes the findings of a quick inspection and the specialist's opinion (were it to be requested) might differ. Dentists tend to see patients in quick succession and many patients (particularly the more anxious ones) might prefer not to spend too long in the dentist's chair. Understandably, a lesion at a very early stage of development might be missed. In contrast, the specialist, with more sophisticated resources and training, should be able to detect problems at an earlier stage. In relying on the check-up, it is important to know how well it compares with the specialist's findings. Methods for assessing this will be discussed in this chapter.

NORMAL RANGE

The term "normal range" is used for the range of a continuous variable (e.g., salivary flow rate) within which we expect measurements for the majority (usually 95% or 90%) of "normal" or disease-free people to be found. It does not mean that the variable has a Normal distribution, but if it does, 95% of the distribution will lie within two standard deviations of the mean (see Chapter 7) or 90% within 1.64 standard deviations. In other words, the 95% normal range is from the mean minus two standard deviations to the mean plus two standard deviations. Note that the term "disease-free" is usually specific to the condition under consideration; it does not necessarily imply that the individual has excellent overall health.

For non-Normal distributions, centiles (sometimes called percentiles) are calculated to estimate the normal range.

Key Message 8.1: Centiles

The 10th centile is the number for which 10% of the data has a lower value, the 5th centile is the number for which 5% of the data has a lower value; the 95th centile has 95% of the data below it and 5% above it. The 50th centile or median is a type of average based on the middle value of the ordered observations.

In order to work out the 95% normal range, the 2.5% and 97.5% points of the distribution would need to be estimated (this would give tails of equal size – 2.5%).

Normal Ranges in Diagnostic Testing

In diagnostic testing, a normal range might be useful if the variable under consideration is continuous. This range would need to be able to distinguish those with the condition from those who do not have it. However, by definition some disease-free people will have a measurement outside the normal range (e.g., 5% outside the 95% range). The degree of overlap between the distribution of values for individuals with a given disease, and the distribution for those without the disease, determines whether or not the measurement is useful for a diagnostic test (Figure 8.1).

In Figure 8.1, the test is determined by fixing a cut-off point above which individuals are provisionally regarded as having the disease, with the remainder being regarded as disease-free. As an example, a

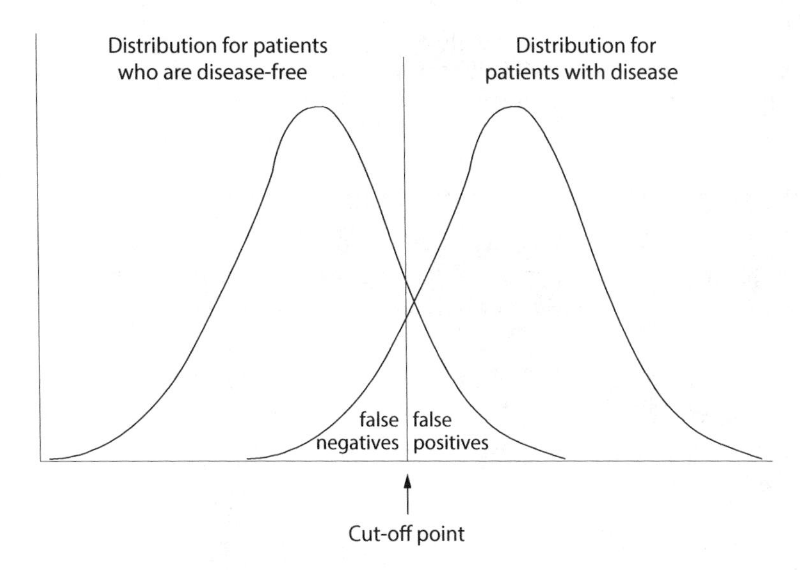

FIGURE 8.1 Using a cut-off point to classify patients as diseased or disease-free.

high level of sugar consumption (typically over 50 g/day) could be a useful indicator of poor dental health. Those who have no significant dental caries but have a high sugar consumption are known as **false positives**; those with poor dental health who have low sugar consumption are known as **false negatives**.

In some situations, a small test value might be diagnostic of the condition (e.g., a low level of iron in the blood indicates the possibility of anemia). In this situation, the positions of the two curves in Figure 8.1 would be interchanged.

> **Key Message 8.2: Moving the Cut-off Point**
>
> By moving the cut-off point, the percentage of false positives can be decreased, but only at the cost of increasing the percentage of false negatives (and vice versa). Few tests achieve perfect discrimination.

This type of testing can sometimes be used to predict those individuals who are at an increased risk of developing a disorder in the future. It may then be possible for high-risk cases to take preventive measures. Diagnostic testing can also be applied if patients can be put into one of two categories following a visual inspection, as in assessing the possibility of oral cancer.

SENSITIVITY AND SPECIFICITY OF DIAGNOSTIC TESTS

Once the variable to be used for the diagnostic test has been identified and the cut-off point has been decided, each individual can be classified as either test positive or test negative. It is important to ascertain:

- ➤ The proportion of individuals with the disease who are accurately classified.
- ➤ The proportion of disease-free individuals who are accurately classified.

The different combinations of diagnostic test result and true disease status in a sample of individuals is shown in Table 8.1.

A laboratory technician would probably be concerned about the **sensitivity** of the test. This is the proportion of individuals out of those with the condition who are detected as having the condition by the diagnostic test:

$$\text{sensitivity} = \frac{\text{the number of diseased individuals positive to the test}}{\text{total number of diseased individuals}}$$

In addition, the **specificity** of the test would be of interest to the technician. This is the proportion of patients out of those without the condition who are detected as not having the condition by the diagnostic test:

$$\text{specificity} = \frac{\text{the number of disease-free individuals negative to the test}}{\text{total number of disease-free individuals}}$$

Key Message 8.3: Measures of Accuracy of the Diagnostic Test

The sensitivity indicates the accuracy with which the test picks up individuals with the disease and the specificity indicates how accurately individuals without the disease are identified.

TABLE 8.1 Screening results and true disease status

	Diseased	*Disease-free*	*Total*
Diagnostic test positive	Number diseased and positive to the test	Number disease-free and positive to the test	Total number of individuals positive to the test
Diagnostic test negative	Number diseased and negative to the test	Number disease-free and negative to the test	Total number of individuals negative to the test
Total	Total number of diseased individuals	Total number of disease-free individuals	Total number of individuals

Note that the definitions of sensitivity and specificity do not depend on the existence of two Normal distributions; they can be calculated as long as the individuals can be divided into two distinct categories (diseased or disease-free).

From the individual's perspective, they are likely to be more concerned about the probability that they have the disease given that they have a positive test result (note that this is not the same as the sensitivity of the test). To answer this question, it is necessary to calculate the **positive predictive value** (PPV):

$$\text{PPV} = \frac{\text{the number of diseased individuals positive to the test}}{\text{total number of individuals positive to the test}}$$

An individual with a negative test result may seek reassurance and wish to know the probability that they are disease-free in the light of their negative diagnosis. The appropriate quantity is the **negative predictive value** (NPV):

$$\text{NPV} = \frac{\text{the number of disease-free individuals negative to the test}}{\text{total number of individuals negative to the test}}$$

These two quantities are more directly relevant to the clinical situation. However, they depend heavily on the true prevalence of the disease in the population. If the disease is relatively rare, the false positives can form a significant proportion of the positive screening results, so the positive predictive value is low despite the sensitivity and specificity being high.

Key Message 8.4: Proportions and Percentages

Note that the sensitivity, specificity, positive predictive value and negative predictive value are frequently presented as the equivalent percentages rather than as proportions.

Example 8.1

A study was conducted into the effectiveness of a brush biopsy as a screening tool for the detection of malignancy in oral mucosal lesions. As part of this investigation, 96 lesions were examined by an OralCDx brush biopsy and by "gold standard" histopathology (Scheifele et al. 2004). For the brush biopsy, lesions were categorized into "positive for dysplasia," "atypical" (less certain), or "negative." The "positive" and "atypical" categories were combined to form the positive screening test group. The results from the screening test and the histological findings are shown in Table 8.2.

The sensitivity of the screening test is the proportion of lesions out of those judged to be malignant on histopathology that had a positive screening result. Of the 26 lesions that were malignant according to histopathology, 24 had a positive screening result. The sensitivity of the screening test is therefore 24/26 (92.3%).

The specificity of the screening test is the proportion of lesions out of those judged not to be malignant according to histopathology that had a negative screening result. Of the 70 lesions that were not malignant according to histopathology, 66 had a negative screening result. The specificity of the screening test is therefore 66/70 (94.3%).

Summary: The test is good for detecting both malignant and non-malignant mucosal lesions.

An individual with a positive screening result based on the lesion examined would be more interested in the probability of true

TABLE 8.2 Screening results and true malignancy status

	Malignant	*Not malignant*	*Total*
Positive screening result	24	4	28
Negative screening result	2	66	68
Total	26	70	96

malignancy (the positive predictive value). Of the 28 lesions with a positive screening result, 24 were malignant according to histopathology. The positive predictive value of the screening test is therefore 24/28 (85.7%).

For an individual with a negative screening result seeking reassurance, the negative predictive value would be useful information. Of the 68 lesions with a negative screening result, 66 were not malignant according to histopathology. The negative predictive value is therefore 66/68 (97.1%).

Summary: The positive predictive value of the screening test is its only weakness, although at 86% it is better than in most diagnostic situations. A few individuals without a malignant oral mucosal lesion will have to undergo worrying further investigations. However, for those with a negative result there is reassuring news. The negative predictive value is excellent, so the risk of having oral cancer based on a single suspicious lesion in this group is tiny.

DECIDING ON THE APPROPRIATE CRITERIA FOR A POSITIVE SCREENING RESULT

In coming to a decision on the appropriate criteria for a positive diagnostic test result it should be noted that changing a cut-off value for a diagnostic test will affect the sensitivity and specificity in opposite directions (see Key Message 8.2). For Example 8.1, consider the likely effect on the sensitivity and specificity of redefining the positive screening group by selecting only those lesions with a "positive" brush biopsy result. By assigning the "atypical" cases to the "negative" group, the number of lesions in the positive screening group will decrease. Fewer genuinely malignant lesions will be detected (the sensitivity will decrease) but by the same token more lesions that are not malignant might be recorded as having a negative screening result (the specificity will increase). Using similar arguments, if the criteria that need to be met for a positive screening result are made less stringent, the sensitivity will increase and the specificity will fall. The authors of the study showed for their data that this is indeed the case.

Example 8.2

For the brush biopsy described in Example 8.1, the sensitivity and specificity values of the screening test were also calculated with the screen positive group consisting only of the "positive" lesions (Table 8.3).

TABLE 8.3 Screening results and true malignancy status

	Malignant	*Not malignant*	*Total*
Positive screening result	16	2	18
Negative screening result	10	68	78
Total	26	70	96

The sensitivity of the screening test is now 16/26 (61.5%), and the specificity is 68/70 (97.1%).

Summary: Using this more demanding definition of a positive screening result gives a much lower value for the sensitivity coupled with barely any increase in the specificity value. With a screening test for cancer that has the potential for a serious diagnosis to be missed, a sensitivity as low as 60% should be avoided where possible. The original broader definition for a positive screening result is therefore more useful as this gives high values for both the sensitivity and the specificity.

The choice of the final criteria will depend on the relative costs to the individual, the health-care system and to society as a whole of a false positive versus a false negative result. For a condition such as oral cancer, in which survival is generally poor and treatment should be commenced as soon as possible, false negative results should be as infrequent as feasibly possible, even if this means that some healthy individuals may have to undergo further investigations. On the other hand, undetected dental cavities are not life-threatening, and routine inspection should be sufficient to avoid serious problems. There are important ethical issues relevant to screening (see Chapter 6).

TEST YOUR UNDERSTANDING

1 Explain what is meant by positive predictive value in the context of screening for dental caries with a probe, against a bite-wing radiograph.
2 What are the likely consequences of a diagnostic test for which unaffected individuals must never receive a positive screening result?
3 A diagnostic study involved the consideration of suspicious oral mucosal lesions by clinical assessment and by "gold standard" histopathology (Güneri et al. 2011). Of the 13 lesions histologically diagnosed with serious pathology, 12 had signs of serious or suspicious pathology on clinical assessment. The 30 lesions that

were found to be benign on histological examination included 17 with indications of serious or suspicious pathology on clinical assessment.

(i) What is meant by the term "gold standard" in this context?
(ii) Define sensitivity and specificity in terms of the above study.
(iii) Indicate the values of the sensitivity and specificity as fractions.
(iv) Comment on the usefulness of the clinical assessment in identifying suspicious oral mucosal lesions and the implications of this for potential patients.

4 A study of young adults investigated the validity of self-reported dental agenesis (DA) using a guided questionnaire. The responses were then compared with childhood dental records and radiographs (Baelum et al. 2011). Of the 176 respondents with documented evidence of DA, 155 (88%) self-reported DA. Of the 117 respondents with no documented evidence of having DA, 110 (94%) reported the absence of DA.

(i) Define sensitivity and specificity in general terms.
(ii) Interpret these definitions in the context of this study.
(iii) This sample was deliberately drawn to include a high proportion of young adults with recorded dental agenesis. If the true prevalence of DA in the population is 7%, what are the implications for self-reported DA as a population-screening tool for the actual occurrence of DA in an individual?

CHAPTER 9

Sampling Variation

INTRODUCTION

The discussion so far has focused on study design and descriptive statistics. In particular, we have seen how a sample can be drawn from a population and looked at some ways in which the data can be presented. Another important aspect of statistics, however, is that of making deductions (inferences) about populations using the information derived from a sample.

To use these methods effectively one should start with a well-defined problem. This needs to be specific, relevant to the investigator's experience, and testable; an oral surgeon is not best placed to investigate neurological changes following the onset of dementia in elderly people. A more appropriate issue might be a comparison of long-term outcome between smokers and non-smokers following the surgical removal of a tumor from the mouth.

A realistic study population of interest needs to be defined (see Chapter 4). It would be inappropriate for an oral surgeon working in London to attempt to make deductions about patients treated in the United States. If the problem under investigation is oral cancer, a suitable study population might be patients with oral carcinoma presenting at the surgeon's place of employment during a particular year. If the oral surgeon is concerned about outcome, a suitable measure might be whether a patient is living one year after the operation. Conclusions should not be drawn from the results of individual patients; an overall summary measure is required for the groups. This might be the proportion of patients alive at one year, calculated for the smoker and non-smoker groups separately. A higher proportion in one of the groups (hopefully the non-smoker group) would indicate a relatively good outcome for that group. If the variable in question were continuous (e.g., systolic blood pressure), the mean could be considered as the summary measure.

It is generally not possible with limited resources in time and money to collect information on all members of the study population. An oral surgeon might only be able to include those patients under his or her direct care; colleagues may not have the time or inclination to be involved. In such a situation, it is important that the sample is as representative as possible of the study population, so enabling the oral surgeon's own patients to be used to generalize about the patients attending the hospital.

The variables must be appropriate and sufficient for the needs of the study, without the collection of irrelevant information. For an oral cancer study, information on smoking is essential. Basic patient information such as age and gender is required, along with lifestyle data such as consumption of alcohol and physical exercise. Possibly irrelevant information that might offend some patients if requested could include issues such as religion and current personal relationships.

The basic statistical methods described in this text require the assumption that within each group the observations are independent of each other. Techniques for dealing with data where the value of one observation can influence the value of another (correlated observations) have been developed but these require a sound background in statistics. Masood, Masood, and Newton (2015) provide an introduction to handling correlated observations in the context of dentistry.

Key Message 9.1: Independence of Individual Observations

Most straightforward statistical methods require the assumption that the observations are independent.

ESTIMATING THE TRUE MEAN IN A POPULATION

Suppose that a dentist is concerned that some of her elderly patients, many of whom have limited financial means, need to travel a considerable distance from their home to her practice in order to receive dental care. This situation might arise in a country where both state and private dental care are available. Typically, some dental practices will treat only private patients, leaving fewer practices available for those who have to rely on state-provided dental care (McKernan et al. 2015).

The dentist decides to conduct a population study into the distances that her elderly patients have to travel to receive their care. She does not have the time available to survey all of these patients and, in any case, since the target population (see Chapter 4) will include future elderly patients as well as those currently registered, it is impossible to include all potential members. A sample of current elderly patients must be selected, and information from the sample used to shed light on what the population is like. For instance, provided the distribution is not too skewed, it is appropriate to use the mean travel distance in a sample as an estimate of the mean travel distance for the population (see Appendix). The sample mean will not in general be exactly the same as the population mean; selecting another sample in the same way will almost certainly yield a different sample mean (see Example 9.1 below).

Key Message 9.2: A Sample Is Just a Guide

The sample mean will only give us an indication as to the value of the population mean. This applies to other sample measurements such as the median, standard deviation, etc.

One might intuitively expect the variation in the means of samples to differ (be smaller?) compared to the variation in the original observations (standard deviation).

Example 9.1
In order to illustrate the relationship between samples and a population, a study population consisting of the 280 elderly patients currently registered on the dentist's list will be considered. The distances travelled, rounded to the nearest mile for convenience, are given below in ascending order (Table 9.1).

TABLE 9.1 Distances (rounded to the nearest mile) from home to dental practice for a population of elderly patients

0	0	0	0	0	0	0	0	0	0	0	0	0	0	0	0	0	0	0	0	1	1	1	1	1	1	1	1	1	1	1	1	1	1	1	1	1	1	1	1
1	1	1	1	1	1	1	1	1	1	2	2	2	2	2	2	2	2	2	2	2	2	2	2	2	2	2	2	2	2	2	2	2	2	2	2	2	2	2	2
2	2	2	2	2	2	2	2	2	2	2	2	2	2	2	2	2	2	2	2	2	2	2	2	2	2	2	2	3	3	3	3	3	3	3	3	3	3	3	3
3	3	3	3	3	3	3	3	3	3	3	3	3	3	3	3	3	3	3	3	3	3	3	3	3	3	3	3	3	3	3	3	3	3	3	3	3	3	3	3
3	3	3	3	3	3	3	3	3	3	3	3	3	3	3	3	3	3	3	3	3	4	4	4	4	4	4	4	4	4	4	4	4	4	4	4	4	4	4	4
4	4	4	4	4	4	4	4	4	4	4	4	4	4	4	4	4	4	4	4	4	4	4	4	4	4	4	4	4	4	4	4	4	4	4	4	4	4	4	5
5	5	5	5	5	5	5	5	5	5	5	5	5	5	5	5	5	5	5	5	5	5	5	6	6	6	6	6	6	6	6	6	6	6	6	7	7	8	8	14

Note that these are illustrative data, as very little has actually been published on the travel distances involved in the receipt of dental care. For this data set, there is a slight positive skew due to the presence of a few outliers and the fact that distances cannot be negative. However, the overall distribution is approximately Normal so it is appropriate to average the data using the mean. For the study population, the mean distance is 2.975 and the standard deviation is 1.717.

How well can a small sample be relied upon to reflect the features of a population? Suppose that 10 random samples of size 5 are selected from this population with distances as follows:

44253	21134	34483	46314	45133
30026	44204	23351	43312	53330

The means for the samples are 3.6, 2.2, 4.4, 3.6, 3.2, 2.2, 2.8, 2.8, 2.6, and 2.8. A sample of this size may give very little insight into the characteristics of the population; the second sample seems to indicate a mean distance of just over two miles whereas the third sample suggests a mean of well over four miles. With this tiny sample size, patients who live close to the practice (those whose travel distance would be rounded down to zero) may be missed altogether or inclusion of the extreme value of 14 miles might raise the sample mean considerably. Despite this, the average sample mean over all 50 observations (3.02) is close to the true mean of 2.975. Within each sample of five patients, the larger and smaller distances tend to cancel each other out. As a consequence, the sample means (2.2 to 4.4) show less variation than the original observations (0 to 14), and the standard deviation of the group means, or **standard error (se)**, (0.689) is much smaller than the overall standard deviation (1.717).

How does the size of the samples selected influence the variation in the group means? To look for a possible relationship, 10 samples of size 10 were taken from the above population of distances. Further groups of 10 samples were taken for the sample sizes 15, 20 and 25. Combined with the findings for samples of size five, the results shown in Table 9.2 were obtained.

As the size of the sample increases, the standard error decreases. In fact, when individual observations are independent of each other, there is a simple theoretical relationship: For the population the standard error is equal to the standard deviation divided by the square root of the group size. This relationship appears plausible from Table 9.2. For the samples of size 25 the standard error is somewhat less than one-half of the standard error for the groups of size 5 and

TABLE 9.2 Sample size and variation in sample means

Size of group	*Standard deviation of group means (standard error)*
Population	1.717 (overall standard deviation)
5	0.689
10	0.596
15	0.556
20	0.463
25	0.271

very roughly one-fifth of the overall standard deviation. With groups as small as these, combined with the selection of only 10 samples per group size, sampling variation can tend to obscure the relationship.

Most studies of dental health in communities use samples of several hundred individuals, so with representative selection the sample means should be close to the true population means.

Key Message 9.3: Sample Size and Standard Error

The greater the number of observations in the sample, the smaller is the standard error of the mean. Large samples from the same population will tend to have similar means.

Consider now the effect of including the extreme distance of 14 miles in one of these samples. For a sample of size five, the mean will be around 3.0 greater than for more typical samples, whereas for a sample of size 25 the increase in the mean, of around 0.5, will be less drastic. Extreme mean values are less frequent as the sample size is increased and the distribution of sample means becomes more symmetrical. Indeed, it approaches the Normal distribution (see Chapter 7); this phenomenon is encapsulated in the Central Limit Theorem (see Appendix, p. 161).

Key Message 9.4: Distribution of Sample Means

The distribution of the sample means is approximately Normal in shape, even when the population distribution is not Normal.

The fact that sample means can often be assumed to be Normally distributed makes them very useful in drawing conclusions about populations.

95% CONFIDENCE INTERVAL FOR A POPULATION MEAN

Once a sample has been collected and the arithmetic mean calculated as an estimate of the population mean, it is important to know whether the estimate from the sample is usually going to be close to the population value (if it is not it will not be of much practical use!). If possible, a range of values should be found within which it is fairly certain that the population mean might lie. A narrow interval would represent a more precise estimate than a wider one.

To keep things simple, assume initially that the population standard deviation of the individual values is known. From the Central Limit Theorem, the sample mean will approximately have a Normal distribution. The standard deviation of the sample means or standard error represents the variation in the values of the sample mean when samples of a particular size are taken. From the properties of a Normal distribution, 95% of the values of the sample mean will be within 1.96 standard errors of the population mean. From this it can be deduced that if an interval is constructed from 1.96 standard errors below the sample mean to 1.96 standard errors above the sample mean, it will contain the population mean with probability of 95% (see Appendix, pp. 161–2).

Key Message 9.5: 95% Confidence Interval

This interval, known as the 95% confidence interval, is one in which there is 95% confidence in the value of the population mean being somewhere within that range.

The value by which the standard error is multiplied in order to obtain a confidence interval is sometimes called the **multiplier**. In the above situation, a multiplier of 2 is sometimes used for convenience instead of 1.96; this gives almost the same answer. Values outside the confidence interval are possible but unlikely. The idea of a 100% confidence interval is appealing, but as this would contain all conceivable values of the population mean it would give no useful information about the most likely values.

Example 9.2

A water company aims to provide a public water supply with a level of fluoride at 1 part per million (ppm). Suppose that water samples are taken at widely spaced times such that the readings can be assumed to be independent of each other. Tests performed on 100 of these water samples give a mean fluoride concentration of 0.85 ppm and an associated 95% confidence interval from 0.76 to 0.94 ppm.

The confidence interval indicates that the best estimate for the population mean is 0.85 and we can be 95% confident that the true mean fluoride concentration is between 0.76 and 0.94 ppm. It is important to remember that this is only a 95% confidence interval. There is still a chance that the true mean could be outside this range. However, the target of 1 ppm fluoride is unlikely to be the true mean as 1.0 lies well outside the confidence interval.

The formula behind the 95% confidence interval used in Example 9.2 can be misleading if there are fewer than around 60 observations. This is because the method is based on the assumption that the true standard deviation is known. In practice, as with the mean, the population standard deviation has to be estimated, in this case by the sample standard deviation (see Example 9.1). With smaller samples this has a noticeable impact, making the true 95% confidence interval a little wider. To compensate for this, the multiplier of 1.96 from the Normal distribution is replaced by a slightly bigger value.

Key Message 9.6: Confidence Interval Width and Sample Size

Wider confidence intervals are obtained with smaller samples because the standard error is larger for smaller samples.

Some assumptions need to be made when using the above method to estimate a population mean and calculate a 95% confidence interval for the population mean.

Key Message 9.7: Assumptions

(a) That the sample is representative of the population.
(b) That the observations are independent of each other.
(c) If the sample size is small, that the variable is Normally distributed in the population.

PAIRED DATA

Paired data have been collected if there are two measurements on the same person or linked measurements on pairs of individuals such as twins. The use of paired data is common in dentistry. For instance, the level of anxiety experienced by patients before and after dental treatment might be of interest. A dentist might want to know whether levels of anxiety decrease or whether they remain broadly the same. It would be necessary to assess the degree of anxiety of the patients at the two time points; each observation before treatment can then be paired with a particular observation after treatment (that of the same patient).

Key Message 9.8: Variable of Interest

For paired data, one is usually interested in the (within-subject) difference between one measurement and the other.

Example 9.3

Many dentists regard tooth enamel as at significant risk of erosion if the salivary pH is below the critical pH value of 5.5 (Dawes 2003). Suppose that a researcher is interested in determining whether use of a leaflet giving dietary advice could influence the salivary buffering capacity pH (a high-sugar intake can increase the acidity of the saliva). Adults identified as being at high risk of future tooth decay were invited to have their salivary buffering capacity measured one week before and one week after receipt of the leaflet. Data from the first 10 participants are shown in Table 9.3.

The researcher would be interested in the difference (within each subject) between salivary buffering capacity before and after receiving the leaflet containing dietary advice. The differences (after – before) have a mean of 0.26 and a 95% confidence interval from 0.105 to 0.415 in salivary buffering capacity pH. This implies that for this population of adults, with 95% confidence the mean increase

TABLE 9.3 Salivary buffering capacity before and after receiving a dietary advice leaflet

Person	*1*	*2*	*3*	*4*	*5*	*6*	*7*	*8*	*9*	*10*
After	5.2	5.5	5.1	5.0	5.6	5.4	5.2	4.9	5.3	5.0
Before	4.9	5.2	5.0	5.1	5.1	4.8	5.0	4.9	4.9	4.7

between salivary buffering capacity after and salivary buffering capacity before the dietary advice is given is between 0.105 and 0.415. An average increase of just over 0.1 is so small as to be of no practical interest; an average increase of 0.4 might be of clinical importance in terms of moving patients vulnerable to further tooth decay to the safe side of the critical pH value. It needs to be borne in mind, however, that not all dentists approve of the rigid use of any critical pH value (Dawes 2003). The views of clinical experts would therefore need to be obtained before taking further action.

95% CONFIDENCE INTERVAL FOR A PROPORTION

Often in dentistry, one of two possible outcomes occurs (e.g., a patient is or is not registered with a dentist; presence or absence of dental caries). The sample is summarized by calculating the proportion with a given outcome (e.g., proportion of the sample with dental caries).

For a sample to give useful information about the population it is necessary to know how close the sample proportion is likely to be to the population proportion. One can estimate a population proportion and calculate a 95% confidence interval for that population proportion in a similar method to that used for the population mean:

- Estimate the population proportion by the sample proportion.
- Calculate the 95% confidence interval from 1.96 standard errors of a proportion below the sample proportion to 1.96 standard errors of a proportion above the sample proportion (for details of calculating this standard error, see Appendix, p. 162).

Example 9.4

In a sample of 80 patients at a dental hospital, 63 of them had been waiting for their treatment for at least three months; in other words, a proportion of $\frac{63}{80}$ or 0.79, with a 95% confidence interval from 0.70 to 0.88.

So, with 95% confidence, we can say that between 70% and 88% of the population of these patients wait for dental treatment for at least three months.

The question "are the findings going to be useful?" should always be asked at the planning stage of a study. Here, the information on waiting times would be useful to administrators, dentists, patients, and politicians (for different reasons!).

Proportions Close to Zero

The method for finding the confidence interval for a proportion described in the Appendix gives only approximate limits. If either of the two possible outcomes is infrequent, so that its proportion is close to zero, the 95% confidence interval calculated by this method may include nonsensical values of less than zero or greater than one. If the number of observations for the less frequent outcome is below five, the exact method based on the binomial distribution should be used (Armitage, Berry, and Matthews 2001). If one of the two outcomes does not occur at all, the lower sample proportion is equal to zero. However, even if a particular outcome is not observed in a sample it does not mean that it can never occur. In fact, the rule of three allows an approximate 95% confidence interval for its true probability to be calculated (Jovanovic and Levey 1997). The lower limit is set at zero (negative values are impossible) and the upper limit is given as 3 divided by the sample size.

Example 9.5

A dentist decides to estimate the proportion of Black Caribbean patients from the first 30 patients treated on a particular day. In the event, no Black Caribbean patients are observed. The sample estimate for the proportion is therefore zero and this is taken as the lower limit of the 95% confidence interval. By the rule of three, the upper limit of the 95% confidence interval is given by $\frac{3}{30}$ or 0.1. Hence the 95% confidence interval for the proportion of Black Caribbean patients is from 0 to 0.1 (this method is reasonable for samples of 30 or more observations; here exact calculation gives an upper limit of 0.095).

Confidence Intervals in Diagnostic Testing

The measures used in diagnostic testing (sensitivity, specificity, and the predictive values) are defined as proportions (Chapter 8). Confidence intervals can therefore be calculated for the measures using the methods for proportions. If a diagnostic test is effective, the sensitivity and specificity values will be close to one, the proportions misclassified will be close to zero, so the exact method based on the binomial distribution should be used.

Example 9.6

In a study of the validity of self-reported dental agenesis (DA) in the identification of true DA (Baelum et al. 2011) the sensitivity of the guided questionnaire used was 0.88, with an associated 95%

confidence interval from 0.82 to 0.92. We can therefore be 95% confident that the true sensitivity of this screening test for DA is between 0.82 and 0.92.

TEST YOUR UNDERSTANDING

1 The standard deviation and standard error are both measures of variation. How do they differ from each other?
2 Explain with an example from dentistry what is meant by the term "paired data."
3 A national chain of chemist stores sells a particular brand of mouthwash. Following a reduction of 10% in the price of the mouthwash, average weekly sales per store rose from 35 to 41 bottles per week, with a 95% confidence interval for the increase from 2.5 to 9.5.
   (i) What information does the confidence interval give about the change in sales?
   (ii) Discuss whether this reduction in price should be extended.

CHAPTER 10

Introduction to Hypothesis Tests

INTRODUCTION

In the previous chapter, we considered how we might obtain a confidence interval for the mean fluoride concentration in a public water supply. As hinted in Example 9.2, there may well be a particular mean value of interest (such as the target mean of 1 ppm fluoride for the water company). This prior idea about the population, which should be stated before the data are collected, is called the **null hypothesis**. Concentration values obtained from water samples by the laboratory are then compared with the claim that has been made about the true mean fluoride level in a process known as testing the null hypothesis.

THE NULL HYPOTHESIS

This initial statement is called the null hypothesis because it is assumed, somewhat cynically, that in a comparison of two groups there is no difference between them in terms of the variable of interest. For example, in an oral cancer study investigating long-term outcome following the removal of a mouth tumor, for the underlying population of patients undergoing surgical removal, the null hypothesis is that the proportion alive at one year is equal for smokers and non-smokers. Without any prior evidence, this makes a natural starting point; the onus is on the investigator to demonstrate to a cynical audience that a difference does indeed exist. Starting from the assumption that the non-smoker group will perform better than the smokers gives the non-smokers an unfair advantage as equivocal results will lead to the conclusion that patients who do not smoke have a better outcome.

The rationale behind the null hypothesis follows the philosophy of Karl Popper, who suggested that most hypotheses can never be proved

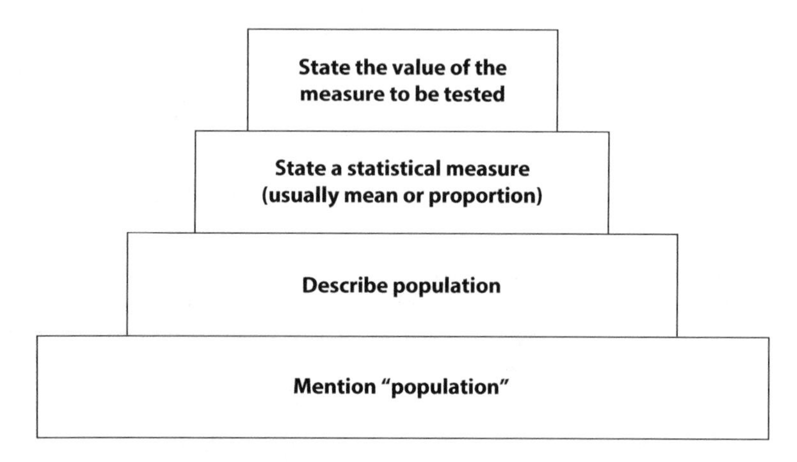

FIGURE 10.1 Constructing a null hypothesis for a single group.

and that knowledge accumulates by the falsification of currently held ideas (Popper 1980). A build-up of evidence against a widely held view eventually leads to it being rejected in favor of an alternative hypothesis, which may in turn be cast aside by future discoveries.

Figure 10.1 shows how a null hypothesis is constructed for a single group. Note that the word **population** is mentioned explicitly in order to emphasize that the null hypothesis refers to the population and not to the sample.

Example 10.1
A suitable null hypothesis for the study of fluoridation levels (Example 9.2) would be that, for the population of potential samples that could be obtained by the water company, the mean level of fluoride is equal to 1 ppm.

Key Message 10.1: Null Hypothesis for One Group

A null hypothesis for one group should include four components: (1) mention 'population'; (2) describe population (e.g. individuals attending a hospital); (3) indicate a summary statistic (e.g. mean or proportion); (4) state value to be tested.

Once the information has been collected, it needs to be analyzed in the light of the null hypothesis. Even if in Example 9.2 the true mean level of fluoride was 1 ppm, it is unlikely that any particular series of water samples would give precisely this value for the mean. Some difference from the true value can be expected just because of random fluctuations between the water samples. How big a difference between the sample mean and the null hypothesis value for the mean (1 ppm) should be allowed before it is reasonable to cast doubt on the null hypothesis? If out of 100 water samples the mean is, say, 0.98 ppm, this does not necessarily indicate much evidence against the null hypothesis. However, what about a sample mean of 0.85 (as in Example 9.2) or 0.70 ppm? In general, the direction of the difference is not of interest, only its size.

For instance, in Example 9.2 (p. 75) a sample mean of 1.15 ppm would be of as much interest as a sample mean of 0.85; the magnitude of the difference is 0.15 ppm in each case. This is what is meant by a "two-tailed test."

Apart from a few exceptions (e.g., if one edentulous individual is found in a village where it has been assumed that everyone has at least some teeth remaining), it is not possible to disprove a null hypothesis, only to say that there is strong evidence against it. Intuitively, the evidence against the null hypothesis should be weak if observed differences from the null hypothesis are small and strong if they are large. The measure that is used to quantify this is known as the *P*-value.

P-VALUES

Key Message 10.2: The *P*-value

The *P*-value is the probability of obtaining at least the difference observed between the sample and null hypothesis values of a measure (e.g., the mean), assuming that the null hypothesis is true. Usually it is the magnitude of the difference (regardless of whether it is positive or negative) that is of concern.

The smaller the *P*-value, the more evidence there is against the null hypothesis. For the case of two groups where the *P*-value is small (e.g., 0.001), under the null hypothesis a difference between the groups of at least the size observed in the sample has a small probability; there is strong evidence against the null hypothesis. For larger *P*-values (e.g., 0.6), the evidence against the null hypothesis is weak because the difference between the two groups is small. It is best to give the exact *P*-value if possible (Figure 10.2).

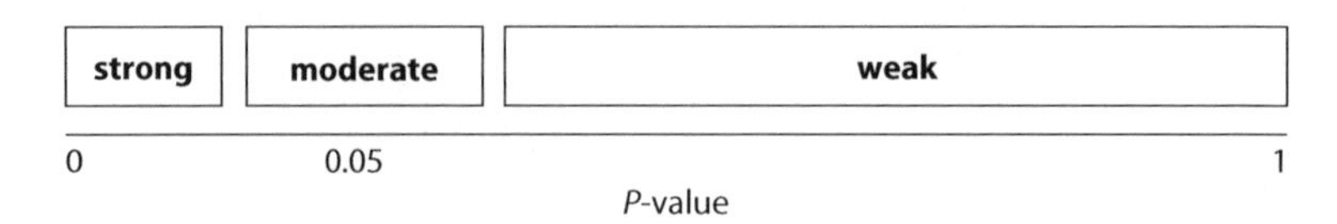

FIGURE 10.2 Strength of evidence (against null hypothesis) interpretation of the *P*-value.

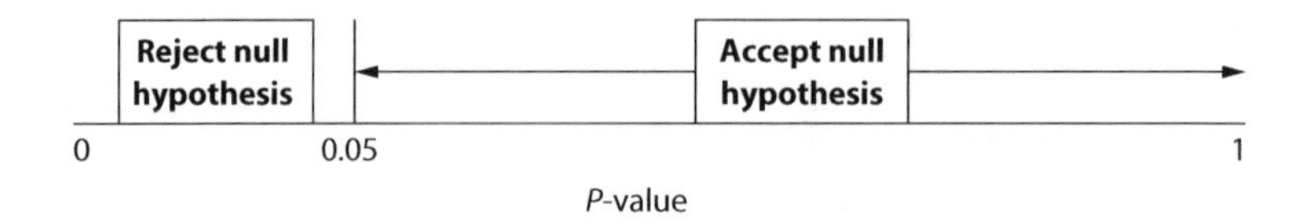

FIGURE 10.3 Traditional interpretation of the *P*-value.

Note when reading dental papers that the traditional interpretation of the *P*-value is sometimes used. This is the convention (used from the 1920s onwards) that the null hypothesis is rejected if $P < 0.05$ and accepted if $P > 0.05$ (Figure 10.3). Such a rigid rule leads to similar *P*-values (e.g., 0.049, 0.051) being interpreted in entirely different ways, which does not make sense! Readers are tempted to conclude (erroneously) that if $P > 0.05$, the null hypothesis must be true.

There is one exception to the usual preference for the strength of evidence interpretation. In the assessment of the size of the sample required for a study (see Chapter 16), the simplistic choice of accepting or rejecting a hypothesis when faced with an alternative hypothesis allows the sample-size calculations to be made in a straightforward way.

Example 10.2

A common misunderstanding is that the *P*-value is the probability of the null hypothesis being true. For a counter-example, consider Figure 10.4. Here a sample with a mean age of 35 years has been drawn from a dental practice population with a mean age of 40 years. Suppose that the null hypothesis is that the mean age in the population for this dental practice is equal to 35 years.

The null hypothesis is certainly false because it is known that the dental practice population mean age and sample mean age differ by five years. However, the sample mean age is equal to the null hypothesis value of 35. The probability that the sample mean differs from the null hypothesis value by at least zero is 1. Using the definition given in Key Message 10.2, the *P*-value is equal to 1. This example therefore demonstrates that a *P*-value of 1 can be obtained even when the null hypothesis (mean = 35) is false (true mean = 40).

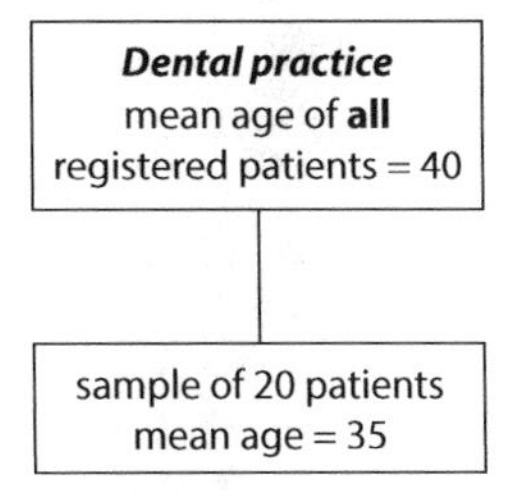

FIGURE 10.4 A *P*-value of 1 does not prove a null hypothesis.

Key Message 10.3: Larger *P*-values

Having a *P*-value close to 1 does not prove that the null hypothesis is true, only that the results are perfectly possible under the null hypothesis.

Further discussion regarding the use of significance tests including the historical context is provided by Sterne and Davey Smith (2001).

Computational Aspects

The traditional method for obtaining *P*-values, used if only a basic electronic calculator is available, is to obtain standard errors and other relevant quantities from the data by hand. A "statistic" is then calculated based on these figures using a formula that is often quite complicated. This calculated value is compared against statistical tables to obtain the appropriate *P*-value (Armitage, Berry, and Matthews 2001). The standard errors are also used in the calculation of the associated confidence intervals. A statistical computer package such as *Stata* will give exact *P*-values and confidence intervals as part of the output from an analysis (StataCorp 2015). Use of a statistical package allows the researcher to concentrate on understanding the principles behind the results and is strongly recommended. For this reason, statistical tables have not been included in this text.

TABLE 10.1 Change in salivary buffering capacity following receipt of a dietary advice leaflet

Person	*1*	*2*	*3*	*4*	*5*	*6*	*7*	*8*	*9*	*10*
Difference	0.3	0.3	0.1	−0.1	0.5	0.6	0.2	0.0	0.4	0.3

An Illustration for Paired Data

Example 10.3

In Example 9.3 the question was whether the use of a leaflet giving dietary advice could influence the salivary buffering capacity pH. For the sample of 10 adults the changes in pH were as shown in Table 10.1.

What value should be chosen for the null hypothesis? The question was: "Does use of the leaflet work?" If the leaflet does not work, there will be no change (on average) between the salivary buffering capacity before and after the leaflet is given. So the population mean change would be 0. To see whether the leaflet works, a true mean change of 0 should be tested.

The null hypothesis is that for the population of adults, the mean change in salivary buffering capacity before and after the leaflet is given is zero.

As found in Example 9.3 the mean change is 0.26. *Stata* shows that the *P*-value – that is, the chance of obtaining a change in the means (positive or negative) of at least 0.26 assuming the null hypothesis is true – is 0.0043. The *P*-value is very small, so there is strong evidence against the null hypothesis. Thus for the population of adults, there is some evidence of a true change between salivary buffering capacity values before and after the leaflet was distributed.

Key Message 10.4: Paired *t*-test

The test described above is known as the paired *t*-test. The data are assumed to be independent observations from a Normal population.

Confidence Intervals and *P*-values

A 95% confidence interval gives the range within which one can be 95% confident about the population mean. Its advantage over a *P*-value is that the values it contains can be assessed relative to those of clinical importance.

> **Key Message 10.5: Position of Null Hypothesis Value with Respect to the 95% Confidence Interval and the Related *P*-value**
>
> If the null hypothesis value is inside the 95% confidence interval, $P > 0.05$; if it is outside the 95% confidence interval, $P < 0.05$. When $P = 0.05$ the null hypothesis value is located at one of the limits of the 95% confidence interval.

However, the actual *P*-value is needed to indicate the strength of the evidence that the sample provides against the null hypothesis.

> **Key Message 10.6: Link between *P*-values and Confidence Intervals**
>
> Carrying out a hypothesis test and finding a *P*-value will lead to the same conclusions about a null hypothesis as calculating a 95% confidence interval and seeing whether the null hypothesis value is inside or outside the confidence interval.

Example 10.4

Compare the result of the hypothesis test ($P = 0.0043$) to the 95% confidence interval calculated in Example 9.3. The null hypothesis value for the mean change, 0, lay outside the 95% confidence interval of 0.105 to 0.415, implying that $P < 0.05$ (Figure 10.5). This agrees with the result of the hypothesis test described above. This sample provides some evidence against the null hypothesis, although as remarked already, the 95% confidence interval might include values of no practical significance (e.g., a possible change in pH of 0.105). Expert opinion would be needed in order to ascertain whether values are large enough to be of clinical importance. Conducting a larger study might be an appropriate way forward (see Chapter 11).

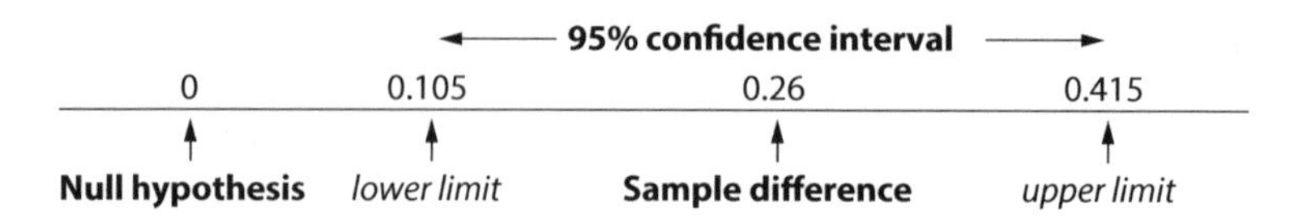

FIGURE 10.5 A 95% confidence interval for the mean change in salivary buffering capacity following receipt of a dietary advice leaflet.

Assumptions Made in Using the Paired *t*-test

The following assumptions are made when a paired *t*-test is applied:

- Observations sampled are representative of the population from which they are selected.
- Differences are all independent of each other.
- Values in one of the two groups can be matched in a one-to-one way to a corresponding value in the second group to form a single set of differences (e.g., "before" and "after").
- Differences come from a population that has a Normal distribution.

The assumption of Normality is only required for small samples. For larger samples (30 or more observations is commonly recommended), substantial deviations from a Normal curve do not make findings from a paired *t*-test particularly misleading.

TEST YOUR UNDERSTANDING

1. A null hypothesis is given as "for the sample of general dental practitioners in New York the mean number of patients treated per day is significantly different from 40." Is this an appropriate statement?
2. Comment on the statement: "If the *P*-value is very small there is strong evidence against the null hypothesis whereas if it is close to 1 there is strong evidence for the null hypothesis."
3. Contrast the role of the value 0.05 in the traditional and strength of evidence interpretations of *P*-values.
4. If a null hypothesis about a population mean is tested, where is the null hypothesis value relative to the 95% confidence interval when the *P*-value is equal to 1?

CHAPTER 11

Comparing Two Means

INTRODUCTION

So far, information from a single sample has been used to make deductions about a population mean using a 95% confidence interval and a hypothesis test. However, often in dentistry two different groups need to be compared on an outcome. For example:

- Do amalgam fillings stay in place longer than composite fillings?
- For privately treated patients, is the mean cost of a crown the same for men and women?
- Is the consultation length (in minutes) of a routine check-up the same for adults with a dental insurance plan as for those without dental insurance?

This chapter looks at how, with two independent samples, a 95% confidence interval for the difference between two population means can be calculated along with a test of the null hypothesis about the difference between those two means.

Key Message 11.1: Difference Between Means

When comparing two populations, we are usually interested in the difference between them. In this case, we are interested in the difference between the two population means.

TABLE 11.1 Length of experience (in years) for a sample of health service and private practice dentists

	Health service	*Private practice*
	1	4
	7	7
	10	8
	13	16
	16	19
	23	23
	25	26
	31	29
	36	32
		37
		41
Number in sample	9	11
Sample mean	18.0	22.0
Sample standard deviation	11.57	12.42

Example 11.1

A local health authority has expressed concern that general dental practitioners are prepared to work for the government health service on qualification but choose private practice once they have gained some professional experience. If this were to be the case, dentists in private practice would on average have longer experience than dentists working for the government health service. For a town within this health authority, the nine dentists working for the government health service and 11 dentists in private practice were asked how many years they had been in practice since qualification (Table 11.1). None of the dentists carried out both health service and private practice work.

The population difference in mean length of experience (private practitioners – health service dentists) is estimated by the observed

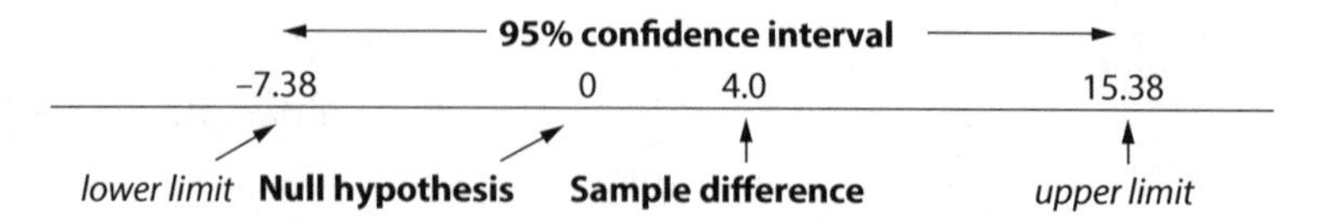

FIGURE 11.1 A 95% confidence interval for the difference between mean length of post-qualification experience (years) between private and health service dentists.

difference in mean length of experience (equal to 4.0 years). The associated 95% confidence interval for the true mean difference can be calculated as being from –7.38 years to 15.38 years. From the principles described in Chapter 9, it can be said with 95% confidence that the population (i.e., true) mean difference between private practice and health service dentists in years of experience is between –7.38 and 15.38. The mean difference in years of experience could be as much as about 15 years more for private practitioners or as much as around seven years more for health service dentists (Figure 11.1).

Differences of seven years or 15 years may be of genuine concern to health service planners and patients. Unfortunately, the 95% confidence interval is so wide that the study did not resolve the original question; the difference in length of experience of dentists could be in either direction. A much larger investigation involving many towns and cities would be required in order to obtain a more accurate estimate of the real differences in years of practice between private and health service dentists.

TWO-SAMPLE HYPOTHESIS TEST

When comparing means from two groups of individuals, the question of interest is usually whether or not the population means are the same; for example, whether mean sugar consumption is greater for females than it is for males. This question is investigated starting from the null hypothesis that there is no true difference and looking for evidence against it.

> **Key Message 11.2: The Null Hypothesis**
>
> A null hypothesis about two independent groups should include five components: (1) mention "population"; (2) describe the population; (3) indicate a summary statistic (e.g. mean or proportion); (4) describe the two groups (e.g., men, women); (5) include "is equal" (Figure 11.2).

Example 11.2

In the study of the length of experience of health service and private practice dentists (Example 11.1), a suitable null hypothesis would be that for the population of dentists practicing in that country, the mean length of post-qualification experience is equal for health service

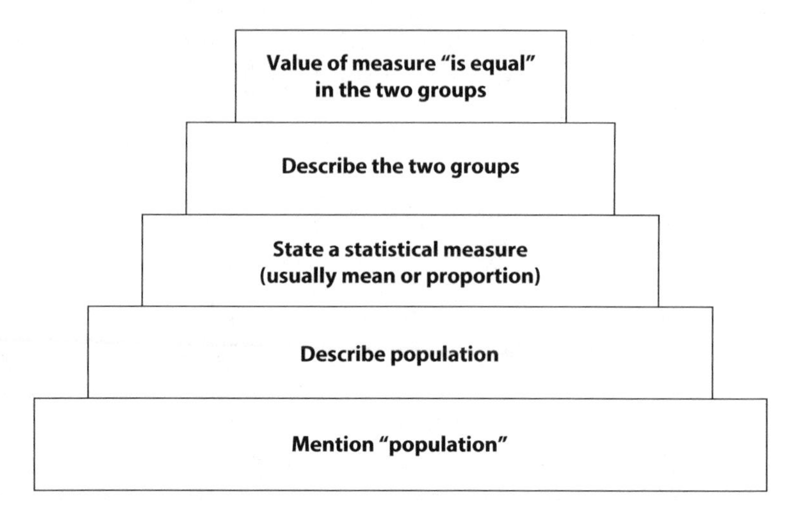

FIGURE 11.2 Constructing a null hypothesis for two independent groups.

and private practice dentists. The sample difference (4 years) for the means gives a *P*-value of 0.470; this can be found by using a statistical package. Since the *P*-value is not small ($P = 0.470$), there is no real evidence against the null hypothesis. Thus there is little evidence that the mean length of experience for the population of dentists is greater for private practice dentists compared to those working in the health service. Remember that a relatively high *P*-value does not prove that the two true means are equal.

Key Message 11.3: Unpaired *t*-test

The test described above is known as the unpaired *t*-test.

Key Message 11.4: *P*-values and 95% Confidence Intervals

It is important to use both a *P*-value and a 95% confidence interval to see whether there is evidence against equality of the two population means, and to examine the clinical relevance for plausible differences.

TABLE 11.2 Implications for a study based on the 95% confidence interval

Null hypothesis value in confidence interval	*Values of clinical importance in confidence interval*	*Implications*
No	All	Change management in light of findings
No	Some	High priority; further studies needed
No	None	Statistically significant differences but unlikely to be of clinical interest
Yes	Some	Lower priority; further studies needed
Yes	None	Any true difference unlikely to be of clinical importance

Clinically Important Values

When a change in treatment or management is under consideration, just demonstrating that the true difference between means is unlikely to be zero is usually not considered to be sufficient. Prior to the study being conducted, the lowest difference required for a change to be implemented is agreed upon; this is sometimes known as the minimum difference for clinical importance. Only if the 95% confidence interval consists totally of values showing clinically important differences is a change in treatment or management made.

The confidence interval may include values that represent a clinically important difference but may also include zero (indicating no evidence against equality of the two population means). On the other hand, the confidence interval may not contain zero, but all the likely values for the difference might be too small to be clinically important. Findings such as these can give unclear messages. Table 11.2 shows the different types of outcome and makes suggestions regarding further research.

Example 11.3

Suppose that in Example 11.1, the minimum clinically important difference in mean ages between the two groups is taken as 5 years. Hence, mean differences (private practice – health service) below –5 years or above 5 years are of clinical interest. The actual 95% confidence interval is from –7.38 to 15.38 years. Hence some of the values are of clinical importance, but the null hypothesis value (0) is also inside the confidence interval. From Table 11.2 the most appropriate action is to conduct further studies.

Assumptions Made in This Test of Means for Two Independent Samples

The following assumptions need to be made when an unpaired *t*-test is applied to two independent groups of observations:

- Each sample is representative of its population. If this is not true, inferences about the populations made from the samples are not valid.
- The observations in the samples are all independent of each other. For example, sampling more than one person from the same family should be avoided.
- The two groups themselves are independent. In particular, the groups should not consist of observations from the same patients taken at two different times (in this case the paired *t*-test might be suitable).
- The data in each underlying population follow a Normal distribution. If sample sizes are around 20 or more, histograms can be drawn and checked for similarities to the "bell-shaped" Normal curve.
- The population variances are equal. This is indicated by the sample variances (square of standard deviations) being similar: The larger sample variance divided by the smaller sample variance should be less than 5.

Where Assumptions Are Not Satisfied

If the distribution of a variable is not Normal, it might be possible to find a transformation that makes it closer to the Normal distribution (e.g., by taking the logarithm of the variable). Care needs to be taken in the choice of transformation. For instance, if the observations include negative values, a logarithmic transformation should not be attempted, as logarithms do not exist for negative numbers.

Other statistical methods that make fewer or different assumptions are available. These can be particularly important if some of the observations are censored; that is, their precise values are unknown but either they exceed a certain value or they are less than a specific value. For censored values, transforming the data is not generally a practical option.

The assumption of Normality is said to be robust for samples with more than about 30 observations; quite large deviations from a Normal curve do not make findings from a *t*-test particularly misleading. However, if sample variances are very different, the results are seriously affected by the breakdown of this assumption. The standard two-sample *t*-test should not be used; a modification of the unpaired *t*-test that allows for unequal variances is available and should be used instead (Armitage, Berry, and Matthews 2001).

TEST YOUR UNDERSTANDING

1 Compare the concepts of strong evidence against the null hypothesis and clinical significance. Is it possible to have one without the other?

2 In a study conducted in the northwest of England, 103 dental practice patients diagnosed with a failed restoration underwent either a replacement or a repair (Javidi, Tickle, and Aggarwal 2015). The findings regarding the time taken by the dentist to complete the intervention were as follows:

	Repair group ($n = 37$)	*Replacement group ($n = 66$)*	P-*value*
Mean time taken (mins)	21.65 (SD 8.02)	25.15 (SD 8.55)	$P = 0.044$

(i) State an appropriate null hypothesis about the time taken to perform the procedure for the two groups.

(ii) Explain the statement "$P = 0.044$". What further information about the difference between the mean procedure times would have improved the presentation of the results?

3 As part of a study of dental anxiety conducted in Chennai, India, 1148 dental hospital outpatients aged 18–70 years completed the Modified Dental Anxiety Scale (MDAS) (Appukutton et al. 2015). A high MDAS score indicates a high level of anxiety about dental treatment. A comparison of the MDAS scores for males and females is given below:

	Males	*Females*
Number of individuals	731	417
Mean MDAS score	10.1	11.1
Standard deviation of MDAS score	3.9	3.9

Difference in mean MDAS score 1.0; *P*-value < 0.001.

(i) State an appropriate null hypothesis for the MDAS score in the two groups.

(ii) The 95% confidence interval for the difference in means (females minus males) is from 0.5 to 1.5. What does this tell us about adult dental outpatients in India?

CHAPTER 12

Dealing with Proportions and Categorical Data

INTRODUCTION

Many outcomes in dentistry are binary (e.g., presence or absence of oral cancer). In Chapter 9 it was seen that a binary outcome in a sample is summarized by calculating the proportion of the sample with a given outcome (e.g., proportion of the sample diagnosed with oral cancer). Dental treatments are often evaluated by comparing a treated group with an untreated (control) group. For instance, the outcome might be the proportions of patients who experienced no pain with new and established anesthetics. If the treatment is "effective," the proportion with the favorable outcome in the treatment group will be higher than that in the control group. Alternatively, we might want to investigate whether people with a high sugar intake are more likely to lose their molars before the age of 65 years compared with people who consume little sugar. If there is no association between sugar intake and loss of molars, the proportion with their molars remaining at 65 years will be the same for those with and without a high sugar intake.

A CAUTIONARY NOTE

This chapter contains examples based on the possible effect of water fluoridation in terms of the development of dental caries. Historically, most published research into the impact of water fluoridation has indicated a benefit in terms of dental caries prevention. However, a recent systematic review of the water fluoridation literature has concluded that a number of factors, such as the use of fluoride toothpaste, diet, and consumption of tap water, need to be considered before water

TABLE 12.1 Evidence of caries in adolescents by type of public water supply

	Non-fluoridated	*Fluoridated*	*Total*
Caries	30 (30%)	24 (20%)	54 (24.5%)
No caries	70 (70%)	96 (80%)	166 (75.5%)
Total	100 (100%)	120 (100%)	220 (100%)

fluoridation is implemented (Iheozor-Ejiofor et al. 2015). The data used here are illustrative so that the explanation is easier to follow; the findings are not intended to reinforce the traditional view. As with all areas of research, dental students and practitioners are advised to keep up to date with current findings.

Example 12.1
A study was conducted into the effect of the fluoridation of the public water supplies on dental caries in adolescence. It was found that 30 out of 100 adolescents (30%) in a non-fluoridated area had evidence of dental caries (indicated by a non-zero DMFT score) compared with 24 out of 120 adolescents (20%) living in a fluoridated area (Table 12.1).

Researchers wanted to know whether adolescents living in areas with fluoridated water supplies are less likely to have caries than those living in non-fluoridated areas: Is the population proportion of adolescents with caries different for those who have fluoridated water from those who do not?

Key Message 12.1: Difference Between Proportions

When comparing two populations, the main concern is usually in the difference between them. Here the interest is in the difference between the two population proportions.

95% CONFIDENCE INTERVAL FOR THE POPULATION DIFFERENCE IN PROPORTIONS

Chapter 9 explains how a 95% confidence interval for the true population proportion is obtained. This confidence interval gives the range of values within which we are 95% confident that the true population proportion lies. To recap, the 95% confidence interval for a population proportion is from 1.96 standard errors of a proportion below the sample proportion to 1.96 standard errors of a proportion above the sample proportion.

In a similar way, the 95% confidence interval for the population difference in proportions is from 1.96 standard errors of the difference in proportions below the sample difference in proportions to 1.96 standard errors of the difference in proportions above the sample difference in proportions (see Appendix, pp. 162–3, for details of how to calculate the standard error of the difference in two proportions).

Example 12.2

For the data in Example 12.1 (fluoridation study) the proportion of adolescents with caries in the non-fluoridated area is 30/100 or 0.3, whereas in the fluoridated area it is 24/120 or 0.2. The observed difference in proportions is therefore 0.1 and this is a reasonable estimate of the true difference in the population. Using the standard error of the difference, calculated to be 0.0586 (see Appendix for details), the 95% confidence interval for the difference in proportions is from −0.015 to 0.215 or −1.5% to 21.5%. We are 95% sure that the population proportion of adolescents with caries is between 1.5% less and 21.5% greater for those from the non-fluoridated area compared to those from the fluoridated area. If the real difference in the proportion with caries were as high as 21.5%, this would strengthen the case for the fluoridation of the public water supply.

However, it is also possible (if unlikely) that the proportion with caries in the non-fluoridated area is slightly less than that in the fluoridated area. The confidence interval here is so wide that it is impossible to make a policy decision based on this study alone.

HYPOTHESIS TEST

When comparing proportions from two groups of individuals, interest is usually focused on whether the population proportions are the same. For example, we might wish to know whether the proportion of adolescents with caries is the same in a fluoridated area as in a non-fluoridated area. As before, we need to establish a null hypothesis and look for evidence against it. This null hypothesis amounts to stating that the two population proportions are the same. As with the comparison of means from two independent groups, the appropriate null hypothesis can be constructed using Figure 11.2.

The strength of the evidence against the null hypothesis will be determined by:

- The size of the difference between the proportions found in the two samples, where a bigger difference leads to stronger evidence.
- The standard error of the difference between the proportions, where a smaller standard error leads to stronger evidence. For any given situation, the standard error decreases as the total sample size increases, so larger samples produce stronger evidence.

As before, the evidence against the null hypothesis is evaluated by carrying out a hypothesis test and calculating a *P*-value.

In order to pursue this further, it is necessary to calculate the difference between the sample proportions divided by the standard error of the difference. The larger the value of this quantity, the lower is the *P*-value and the stronger the evidence against the null hypothesis. The standard error for the difference in proportions is not the same as that in the calculation of the corresponding confidence interval in Example 12.2, because the null hypothesis is assumed to be true (usually this leads to a slight but inconsequential difference in the two values). Details of how to calculate the standard error for the difference in proportions in this case are given in the Appendix (p. 163).

Example 12.3

Using the data from Example 12.1, the null hypothesis is that in the population of adolescents, the proportion with caries is equal in the fluoridated and non-fluoridated areas. The difference in proportions of 0.1 along with the standard error of the difference, which is 0.0583 (details of this calculation are in the Appendix; see p. 163) gives a ratio that implies that the *P*-value is 0.086. The *P*-value is not particularly small so there is not a lot of evidence against the null hypothesis. Therefore, there is little evidence (from this study alone) that adolescents from areas with fluoridated water are less likely to experience caries.

Key Message 12.2: Test of Two Independent Proportions

The test described above is known as the test of two independent proportions.

THE CHI-SQUARED TEST

This is an alternative method for testing the null hypothesis that two population proportions are equal. The *P*-value obtained using the chi-squared test is exactly the same as that obtained using the method described above. The chi-squared test looks at the difference between the number of people in each cell of the table, and the number anticipated were the null hypothesis to be true (details of the calculation of the expected values are given in the Appendix; see p. 164). A quantity based on the differences between the observed and expected values, known as the chi-squared statistic, is then calculated. If the observed numbers in each entry of the table are exactly as expected from the null hypothesis, this statistic is zero.

> **Key Message 12.3: Interpreting the Chi-Squared Statistic**
>
> The bigger the value of the chi-squared statistic, the further the observed data are from those expected from the null hypothesis, the smaller is the *P*-value and the stronger the evidence against the null hypothesis.

Note that the chi-squared test has no directly associated confidence interval.

Example 12.4

For the data from the fluoridation study (Example 12.1) the chi-squared statistic is 2.945 (for details of this calculation, see Appendix, p. 165) and the *P*-value is equal to 0.086. This *P*-value is not particularly small, indicating that the sample provides no clear evidence against the null hypothesis. From this fairly small study, it is perfectly feasible that the proportion of adolescents with caries is the same in fluoridated and non-fluoridated areas.

Variables with More Than Two Categories

The main advantage of the chi-squared test is that it can be applied to larger tables where there are more than two rows and two columns. A variable may well have more than two response categories, particularly where degrees of health or attitudes of individuals are concerned.

TABLE 12.2 Observation of any arrhythmia and the anesthetic used in the extraction

	Halothane	*Incremental sevoflurane*	*8% sevoflurane*	*Total*
Any arrhythmia	24 (48%)	4 (8%)	8 (16%)	36 (24%)
No arrhythmias	26 (52%)	46 (92%)	42 (84%)	114 (76%)
Total	50 (100%)	50 (100%)	50 (100%)	150 (100%)

Example 12.5

There has been some concern that the use of general anesthesia for children having dental surgery can produce arrhythmias (deviations from the normal rhythm of the heart) and that halothane may be more likely to produce these than some other anesthetics. To investigate this occurence, 150 children between three and 15 years of age having dental extractions performed under general anesthesia were randomly allocated either to halothane, incremental sevoflurane, or 8% sevoflurane (Blayney, Malins, and Cooper 1999). The results for the production of any arrhythmia were as shown in Table 12.2.

The null hypothesis is that in the population of children having dental extractions under general anesthesia the proportion of children experiencing arrhythmias is the same, irrespective of the anesthetic used in the extraction. Under the null hypothesis an expected value can be calculated for each cell from the corresponding row total and column total, and in the chi-squared test these expected values are compared with the observed values shown in the above table.

The value of the chi-squared statistic is 24.56 (for details see the Appendix, pp. 165–6). This is equivalent to a *P*-value of much less than 0.001. Since the *P*-value is tiny there is strong evidence against the null hypothesis. Thus there is real evidence that in the population of children having dental extractions under general anesthetic, the proportion of children experiencing arrhythmias differs depending on the anesthetic and that halothane is particularly risky. It is highly unlikely that such a result would have occurred by chance had the anesthetics all been truly of equal risk for producing arrhythmias.

Degrees of Freedom

In both Examples 12.4 and 12.5 it was stated that the higher the value produced by the chi-squared test calculation, the lower the corresponding *P*-value. There is a further twist to this – if two tables of different sizes produce the same chi-squared statistic, the larger table will have the larger corresponding *P*-value. For instance, in Example 12.4 (a table with two rows and two columns – see p. 98), a chi-squared statistic of 2.945 corresponds to a *P*-value of 0.086. Had the table in Example 12.5 (with two rows and three columns) produced the same chi-squared statistic of 2.945, the corresponding *P*-value would have been 0.2294. In other words, a larger table needs to produce a greater chi-squared statistic in order to have a *P*-value that corresponds to strong evidence against the null hypothesis. A table with two rows and two columns needs a chi-squared statistic of 3.84 for a *P*-value of 0.05, whereas one with two rows and three columns needs a chi-squared statistic of 5.99 for the same *P*-value.

Why might this be? It comes down to what is known as the **number of degrees of freedom**. In a table with two rows and two columns, it might seem that the four inner cells are free to take any value. However, if the row and column totals are known (which they must be for studies such as Example 12.1), once the value of a single inner cell is known the other three values can be deduced by subtraction from these totals, as in Example 12.1 (Table 12.3).

So the above table has just **one** degree of freedom, not four. Similarly, there are only two degrees of freedom (not six) in Example 12.5 (Table 12.4).

TABLE 12.3 Only one cell value is needed in order to fill in the other three cells

	Non-fluoridated	*Fluoridated*	*Total*
Caries	**30**	*24*	**54**
No caries	*70*	*96*	**166**
Total	**100**	**120**	**220**

Bold: Cell value known; italic: Cell value deduced.

TABLE 12.4 Only two cell values are needed in order to fill in the other four cells

	Halothane	*Incremental sevoflurane*	*8% sevoflurane*	*Total*
Any arrhythmia	**24**	**4**	*8*	**36**
No arrhythmias	*26*	*46*	*42*	**114**
Total	**50**	**50**	**50**	**150**

Bold: Cell value known; italic: Cell value deduced.

In general, the number of degrees of freedom is equal to one less than the number of rows multiplied by one less than the number of columns.

SMALL SAMPLES

If the total number of observations in a table is small, particularly if some of the categories occur infrequently, the chi-squared test can give misleading conclusions. An oft-quoted rule is that ignoring row and column totals, every entry in the table should have an expected value of at least 1 and for at least 80% of the entries the expected value should be at least 5 (Armitage, Berry, and Matthews 2001). So, for a table with two rows and two columns, no expected value should be less than 5. The expected value requirement is met if the observed frequency of each cell is at least 5; it is sometimes true if the smallest observed frequency is less than 5, as in Example 12.5, where the smallest observed value is 4 (see Table 12.2) but the smallest expected value is 12 (see Appendix, p. 166). If the sample is small, categories can be amalgamated to produce larger expected values. If this cannot be achieved in a meaningful way, Fisher's exact test can be used instead (Armitage, Berry, and Matthews 2001). This test is available on some statistical computer packages, such as *Stata* (StataCorp 2015). The *P*-value obtained by this method provides a reliable interpretation of the data.

TEST YOUR UNDERSTANDING

1 Determine the number of degrees of freedom in a table having three rows and four columns.
2 The following 95% confidence intervals represent the difference in the percentage with gingivitis in a comparison of male and female young adults. The null hypothesis is that the true percentages are equal for males and females. Suppose that a difference in percentages of 5% is of clinical importance. Match the inferences (i–v) with the options (a–e).

   Options for male percentage minus female percentage (↔ denotes confidence interval):

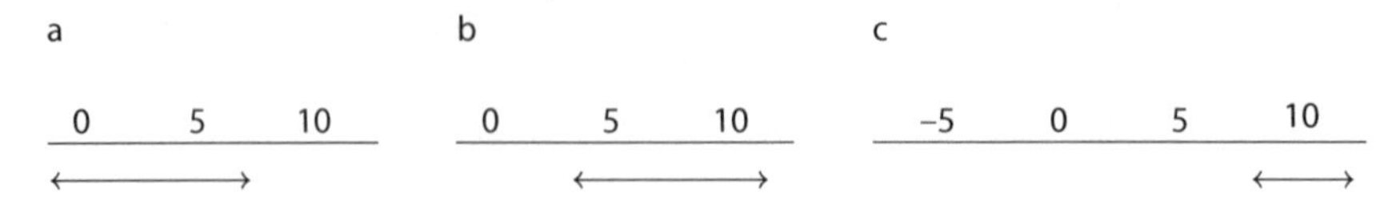

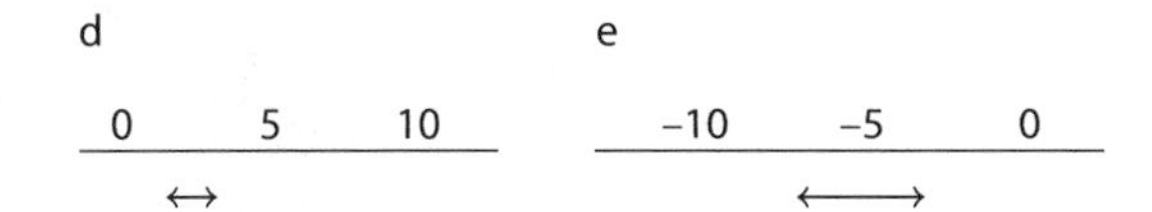

(i) Evidence that a greater percentage of females have gingivitis
(ii) Strong evidence that a greater percentage of males have gingivitis – all values within the confidence interval are of clinical importance
(iii) The *P*-value is slightly greater than 0.05
(iv) No differences within the confidence interval are of clinical importance
(v) The null hypothesis is plausible.

3 In a study of the attitudes in the American dental profession towards the Medicaid scheme for affordable care targeted at those with a low income, 651 dentists based in Iowa were asked whether they currently accepted new Medicaid patients into their practice (McKernan et al. 2015). A comparison of those living in a metropolitan county of Iowa with those living in a non-metropolitan county gave the following results:

	Metropolitan	*Non-metropolitan*
Number of dentists	371	280
Number accepting new Medicaid patients	194	172
Percentage accepting new Medicaid patients	52.3%	61.4%

Difference in percentage accepting new Medicaid patients (non-metropolitan – metropolitan) = 9.1% (two significant figures), 95% confidence interval for difference 1.4% to 16.8%, $P = 0.02$.

(i) State an appropriate null hypothesis for the acceptance of new Medicaid patients by metropolitan and non-metropolitan dentists in Iowa.
(ii) What does the 95% confidence interval indicate about the willingness of metropolitan and non-metropolitan dentists to accept new Medicaid patients?

CHAPTER 13

Comparing Several Means

INTRODUCTION

In Chapter 11 we considered the comparison of means from two independent groups, and the comparison of two proportions was explained in Chapter 12. The previous chapter also showed how the chi-squared test for two-way tables can be extended to the case of comparing proportions from three or more groups. This raises the question of how means from three or more independent groups can be compared, the subject now to be addressed.

Examples of research questions for which the mean might be suitable in a comparison of several groups include:

- Is the length of time spent examining a patient the same, on average, for several dentists working within the same practice?
- Is the number of registered patients per dental practice similar for socioeconomically affluent, intermediate, and deprived districts in the United States?
- Is the average cost of a crown the same for adult private patients living in England, Scotland, and Wales?

This chapter describes one-way analysis of variance (ANOVA) as applied to several independent groups. The method is an extension of the unpaired *t*-test and the calculations involved with one-way ANOVA reduce to those for the unpaired *t*-test when the number of groups is equal to two. The rationale behind the method will be covered here; the algebraic details of ANOVA can be found elsewhere (Armitage, Berry, and Matthews 2001). The illustrative examples used in this chapter relate to an extension of the mouth rinse Case Study discussed in Chapter 5.

CASE STUDY EXTENSION: ASSESSING PATIENT RECRUITMENT

Following the promising investigation by Mary Williams, a larger study of Xellent and Ynot is funded, to be based in the UK. The dental practitioners involved in the Birmingham area are Mary Williams and four other local dentists; the local study coordinator is Mary's former dental public health tutor, Jon. Each dentist has been asked to recruit at least five appropriate patients per working day. After three weeks, Jon checks on the numbers of patients recruited on each day by the Birmingham dentists and obtains the information presented in Table 13.1.

Example 13.1

Jon uses the information from the first three weeks to check that the dentists are meeting the daily rate for target patient recruitment. Table 13.1 shows that on average all the dentists are meeting the target of five patients per day. David, Gareth, and Tara have had occasional days on which the target has not been met but overall the situation is satisfactory. Mary appears to be more successful at recruiting patients,

TABLE 13.1 Daily recruitment of patients to the mouth rinse study for each of the participating dentists

	Anand	*David*	*Gareth*	*Mary*	*Tara*
	5	4	5	7	8
	7	6	4	8	6
	8	7	6	9	6
	8	7	7	8	8
	7	6	3	8	6
	9	8	5	10	9
	5	4	6	5	5
	6	6	8	8	7
	5	4	6	6	6
	9	7	4	10	4
	7	6	6	7	
	7	6	5	9	
	6	5	5	7	
	6	5	7	7	
	7	6		8	
Number in sample	15	15	14	15	10
Sample mean	6.8	5.8	5.5	7.8	6.5
Sample standard deviation	1.32	1.21	1.34	1.37	1.51

although daily random fluctuation might be the simple explanation. An appropriate hypothesis test is required to explore this further. For simplicity, the observations within each of the five groups are assumed to be independent (this would not necessarily be the case in practice).

Multi-sample Hypothesis Test

When comparing means from several groups of individuals, the question of interest is usually about whether the population means are the same. The investigator starts with the null hypothesis that there is no true difference between the means and then looks for evidence against it. For the mouth rinse study, these means refer to the average daily number of patients recruited by each dentist.

Key Message 13.1: Difference Between Means from Several Groups

When comparing several populations, we are initially interested in whether there are any **differences** between population means overall.

If there is evidence against the null hypothesis showing that the population means are likely to differ, it may be useful then to look at the differences between pairs of groups. If there is no evidence against the null hypothesis, this finding should be reported but individual pairs of groups should not be inspected.

Key Message 13.2: The Null Hypothesis

A null hypothesis about several independent groups should include five components: (1) mention "population"; (2) describe the population; (3) indicate a summary measure (e.g. mean or proportion); (4) describe the groups (e.g., socioeconomically affluent, intermediate, deprived); (5) mention that the value of the measure "is equal" across the groups.

Note that Figure 11.2 requires only minor rewording for use with the construction of multi-sample null hypotheses.

Example 13.2
For the mouth rinse study, a suitable null hypothesis would be that the population mean number of patients recruited daily is equal for each of the five participating dentists. In fact, the sample means range between 5.5 and 7.8. One-way analysis of variance gives a very small P-value ($P < 0.001$).

Since the P-value is so small, there is strong evidence against the null hypothesis. Thus there is strong evidence that the true mean number of patients recruited daily differs between the five dentists. Gareth and David may genuinely have been recruiting at a lower rate than Mary in the long term.

Clinically Important Values

As with two groups, it is not sufficient just to demonstrate that the true difference between means is unlikely to be zero. The differences highlighted should also be of clinical importance before a change in management is made. If the differences presented in Table 13.1 are important it might be helpful for Jon to organize a meeting with Mary, who has experienced previous practice-based research and appears to be recruiting effectively, and the other participating dentists. If the differences are not of practical importance it might be better for Jon simply to continue his monitoring of the recruitment.

Assumptions Made in Using One-Way Analysis of Variance for Several Independent Samples

The following assumptions need to be made if one-way ANOVA is applied to independent groups of observations:

- Each sample is representative of its population. If this is not true, inferences about the populations made from the samples are not valid.
- The observations in the samples are all independent of each other. For example, sampling more than one person from the same family should be avoided.
- The groups themselves are independent. In particular, the groups should not consist of observations from the same patients taken at different times (e.g., one day, one week, two weeks after a procedure).
- The data in each underlying population follow a Normal distribution. If sample sizes are around 20 or more, histograms can be drawn and checked for similarities to the "bell-shaped" Normal curve.

- The population variances are equal. This is indicated by the sample variances (square of standard deviations) being similar. It is impossible to give a watertight rule but most sources recommend that for this assumption to be entertained, the largest sample variance divided by the smallest sample variance should definitely be less than 4.

Note that as with the paired and unpaired *t*-tests, the population Normality assumption is only important if some of the groups have only a small number of observations.

Examining Pairs of Groups Following a Multi-Sample Hypothesis Test

If the overall hypothesis test (one-way ANOVA) shows evidence against the null hypothesis, it may be appropriate to identify the groups most likely to be responsible for the differences between the means. One way of approaching this is to analyze each pair of groups in turn using the unpaired *t*-test. It might be concluded that the pairs of groups showing evidence against equal population means are responsible for the evidence against the overall ANOVA hypothesis.

> **Key Message 13.3: *Post-hoc* Testing of Pairs of Groups**
>
> The analysis of pairs of groups subsequent to the initial one-way analysis of variance being performed is sometimes described as *post-hoc* testing. It should only be carried out if there is evidence against the multi-sample null hypothesis.

There are two important points to consider when applying *P*-values to *post-hoc* testing. Firstly, although the subjective approach to *P*-value interpretation is preferable when just one null hypothesis is being considered, in the *post-hoc* testing of pairs of groups a fairly traditional interpretation of the *P*-value is taken. This is really just to be practical, as sliding scales of strength of evidence do not provide a clear overall picture when many hypotheses are being examined together. More importantly, the *P*-values themselves need to be adjusted to take into account the fact that several null hypotheses are being tested together. Suppose that pairs of groups are tested in turn and we decide that for each null hypothesis there is reasonable evidence against it being true if the *P*-value is less than 0.05. Assume that the overall null hypothesis (equal population means across all of the groups) is in fact true. Then for each pair of groups the corresponding null hypothesis (that the two population means are equal) is also true. Taking the first pair of groups, the probability of not finding evidence against its null hypothesis is therefore 1 minus 0.05 or 0.95. For the second pair, this probability is also equal to 0.95. Hence there is a probability of 0.95 × 0.95 or roughly 0.9 of finding no evidence against both of these two pairwise null hypotheses. This finding can be expressed alternatively as a probability of around 2 × 0.05 of incorrectly reporting some evidence against at least one of the two pairwise null hypotheses. By the same logic, for three pairs of groups the probability of seeing some evidence against at least one of the three pairwise null hypotheses is approximately 3 × 0.05 or 0.15. In general, the chance of seeing some evidence against at least one of the pairwise null hypotheses increases with the number of pairs involved, eventually leading to the situation whereby it would be surprising *not* to see any "significant" pairwise results.

Example 13.3

The dentists involved (A, D, G, M, T) are to be compared in pairs. There are 10 possible matches (AD, AG, AM, AT, DG, DM, DT, GM, GT, MT). Suppose that for each pair, $P < 0.05$ is taken as sufficient evidence for rejecting the pairwise null hypothesis. The probability of finding evidence against a correct null hypothesis for Anand and David is therefore 0.05; the same is the case for the other pairings. Taking all 10 pairings together, a first guess for the probability of seeing some evidence against at least one of the null hypotheses is 10 × 0.05 = 0.5 or about a 50:50 chance (a more detailed and accurate calculation is given in the Appendix). Hence, it is easy to discover pairings with apparently "significant" differences even though the initial null hypothesis of the equality of all population means is true.

Key Message 13.4: Simultaneous Testing of Null Hypotheses

If several groups are compared by considering pairs of groups in turn, there is a high probability of finding evidence against at least one of the null hypotheses even if the initial null hypothesis that all of the population means are equal is true.

THE BONFERRONI CORRECTION

As seen already, multiplying the number of pairwise comparisons by the null hypothesis rejection *P*-value (customarily 0.05) can, for small numbers of pairs, give a reasonable first guess for the probability of seeing some evidence against at least one of the null hypotheses. The Bonferroni correction applies this logic in reverse. It states that the *P*-value to be used in interpreting the results for individual pairwise analyses should be set equal to the *P*-value applied in the initial overall hypothesis test divided by the number of pairwise comparisons made in the *post-hoc* testing.

Example 13.4

For the mouth rinse study, the use of a *P*-value of less than 0.05 to indicate sufficient evidence against each pairwise null hypothesis gives very roughly a tenfold probability of seeing some evidence against at least one of the null hypotheses in *post-hoc* testing that involves all five groups. Applying the Bonferroni correction, the probability of seeing some evidence against at least one of the pairwise null hypotheses at the *post-hoc* stage will be reduced to around 0.05 if the *P*-value used for specific pairs is set equal to 0.05/10 or 0.005.

Testing each pair of groups in turn without regard to the other pairings can have serious implications for the conclusions drawn, as shown below.

TABLE 13.2 Findings for the unpaired *t*-test comparisons of the pairs of participating dentists on the mean number of patients recruited per day (a) without and (b) with the Bonferroni correction

	Difference in means	*95% confidence interval*	P-*value*	*(a)* P < *0.05*	*(b)* P < *0.005*
Anand vs. David	1.0	0.05 to 1.95	0.039	Yes	No
Anand vs. Gareth	1.3	0.28 to 2.32	0.014	Yes	No
Anand vs. Mary	-1.0	-2.01 to 0.01	0.052	No	No
Anand vs. Tara	0.3	-0.88 to 1.48	0.600	No	No
David vs. Gareth	0.3	-0.67 to 1.27	0.532	No	No
David vs. Mary	-2.0	-2.97 to -1.03	<0.001	Yes	Yes
David vs. Tara	-0.7	-1.83 to 0.43	0.211	No	No
Gareth vs. Mary	-2.3	-3.34 to -1.26	<0.001	Yes	Yes
Gareth vs. Tara	-1.0	-2.21 to 0.21	0.102	No	No
Mary vs. Tara	1.3	0.09 to 2.51	0.036	Yes	No

Use of $P < 0.05$ for individual pairs gives evidence against the null hypothesis for five of the comparisons, with a suggestion of some evidence against the null hypothesis for Anand vs. Mary. If the Bonferroni correction is applied, there is only evidence against the pairwise null hypotheses for David vs. Mary and Gareth vs. Mary. With the correct analysis only Mary seems to be recruiting at a genuinely higher rate.

A Weakness of the Bonferroni Correction

In Example 13.4, adjusting the pairwise P-values in the manner indicated by the Bonferroni correction does not lead to the intended probability of seeing some evidence against at least one of the null hypotheses being exactly equal to 0.05. The true probability is somewhat less, at around 0.049 (the calculation is given in the Appendix). This is because the Bonferroni correction is based on a simple approximation to a rather more complicated algebraic formula. Although the difference might seem small in this example, in some situations the discrepancy can be appreciable. The Bonferroni correction should therefore be applied with this caution in mind.

Other methods of adjusting for multiple testing using pairs of groups have been developed (Armitage, Berry, and Matthews 2001) and the choice of the most appropriate technique should be discussed with a statistician.

TEST YOUR UNDERSTANDING

1 Consider the assumptions made in using one-way analysis of variance, listed in the options. For each of the scenarios described below, select the assumption that is most obviously untrue.

Options:

(a) Each sample is representative of its population.
(b) Within each sample observations are independent of each other.
(c) Observations in one sample are independent of observations in the others.
(d) Observations in each population follow a Normal distribution.
(e) The population variances are equal.

Scenarios:

(i) Dental health education sessions were held (a) at a school year-group meeting (b) in a whole-school meeting (c) at a local community centre. The ages of those attending (excluding teachers for the schools) were obtained. For the year-group meeting the mean was 12 and the standard deviation was 0.25, for the whole-school group the mean was 15 and the standard deviation was 1.5, and for the community centre group the mean was 40 and the standard deviation was 10. The three groups are to be compared on age.

(ii) Information is required about the use of toothpaste and floss by children living in Britain. The samples are drawn from children admitted to British dental hospitals.

(iii) Adults from England, Scotland, and Wales were compared on the number of cigarettes smoked per day. The three samples included non-smokers.

(iv) The five samples consist of measurements of salivary flow rate taken on the same individuals and obtained on five consecutive days.

(v) Samples were taken that included all of the children living in selected households.

2 An investigation was conducted on patients aged less than 21 regarding who, if anyone, accompanied them to their appointment at a dental hospital (family member, a friend, attended alone). The findings regarding the mean age for each group were:

With family member	*With friend*	*Alone*	P-*value*
10.2	18.1	19.5	<0.001

(i) State an appropriate null hypothesis about the mean age of the patients in the three groups.

(ii) Explain the statement "$P < 0.001$".

(iii) What further testing could be performed between the three groups?

(iv) Why might the values of the means shown above cast doubt on the assumptions involved in applying one-way analysis of variance to these data?

CHAPTER 14

Regression, Correlation, and Agreement

INTRODUCTION

When the relationship between two continuous variables is explored, the first stage should be to construct a **scatter diagram**. Figure 14.1 is such a diagram, illustrating the relationship between home to dental practice distance and income for a group of young adults. Once a graph has been obtained, regression and correlation can be used to describe the relationship numerically.

REGRESSION

The process of describing a mathematical relationship between two or more quantitative variables is known as regression. In its simplest form, regression can be used to fit a straight line between two continuous variables.

Example 14.1

Suppose that the question of interest is whether the distance from home to dental practice is influenced by annual income for young adults. Some dental practices treat only private patients, leaving fewer practices available for those who have to rely on state provision (McKernan et al. 2015). Less well-off adults might therefore have to travel further to receive their dental care and there is some evidence from the United States that this is indeed the case (Probst et al. 2007). Using illustrative data, a scatter diagram has been plotted in which the outcome variable (travel distance in miles) is on the vertical axis and the explanatory variable (annual income in £K) is on the horizontal

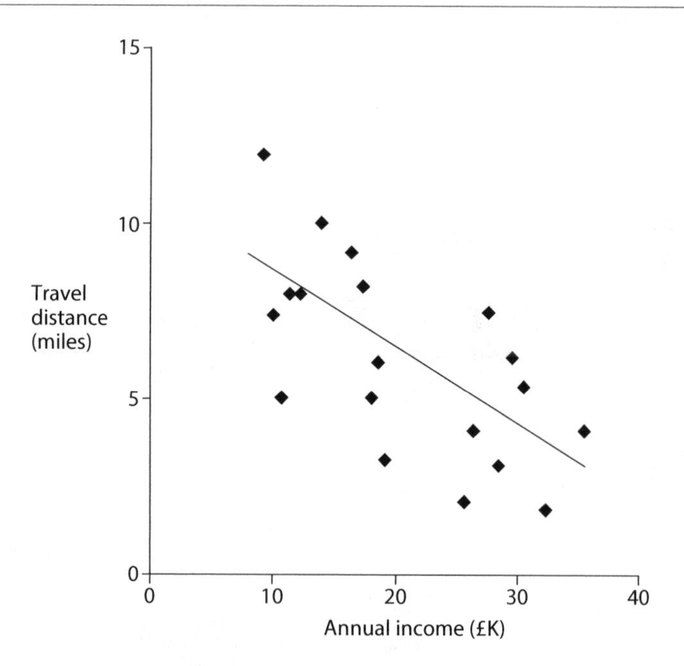

FIGURE 14.1 Scatter diagram showing home to dental practice travel distance against income for a group of young adults.

axis for a group of registered patients living in a socially disadvantaged rural area (Figure 14.1).

Looking at Figure 14.1 it can be seen that there is a general relationship between travel distance and income in £K and that the data appear to be scattered around a straight downward-sloping line. Such a relationship is called a **linear association**. In other words, it is assumed that when the explanatory variable increases by a given amount, there is a corresponding (average) increase or decrease in the outcome. Linear regression is used to predict the value of the outcome variable (travel distance) for a given value of the explanatory variable (annual income).

Key Message 14.1: Linear Regression

Linear regression is used to investigate a straight line (linear) association between two quantitative variables; the straight line that is fitted to the scatter diagram is known as the regression equation.

Describing a Straight Line

In linear regression we estimate the gradient for the "best" straight line that describes the relationship between the variables. In addition, in order to fix the position of the line it is necessary to know the value of the outcome variable (e.g., distance) predicted by the line when the explanatory variable (e.g., annual income) is zero. The gradient of the slope can be referred to as the regression coefficient. The predicted travel distance for zero income – the point where the regression line meets the vertical axis – is known as the intercept. In Figure 14.1, the gradient represents the (negative) difference in travel distance (on average) for each additional £1000 in annual income.

Least Squares

Whatever the choice of regression line, most if not all of the points will lie away from the line – implying that there are errors between the observed and predicted travel distances for particular incomes. Since it is difficult to choose an appropriate regression line simply by inspecting the scatter diagram, a regression line is generally fitted using a computer by a mathematical method known as **least squares**. The regression line in Figure 14.1 was fitted in this way. In the least squares method, the sum of the squared discrepancies between the observed and predicted values is minimized. This method is reasonable since it seeks to avoid relatively large errors; these are penalized heavily because their squared values considerably inflate the overall sum.

Example 14.2

For the scatter diagram in Example 14.1 the gradient (regression coefficient) is –0.22 (i.e., on average the travel distance will be less by 0.22 miles for each increase of £1000 in income) and the predicted travel distance for zero income is 10.82 (this implies that on average within this area young adults with little income, e.g., the unemployed, need to travel further for dental care).

Once a regression line has been fitted, it is important to investigate whether the relationship between the two variables is genuine or whether it might be due to chance.

Key Message 14.2: Null Hypothesis for Linear Regression

If the two variables are independent of each other, the true gradient of the regression line between them (regression coefficient) is zero. The corresponding null hypothesis is that in the population from which the sample was taken, the regression coefficient is zero.

Example 14.3

In Example 14.1, the null hypothesis is that for the population of young adults, the regression coefficient (slope) for travel distance against annual income is zero (i.e., there is no relationship between travel distance and annual income).

In a similar way to the analyses discussed in previous chapters, we can calculate a 95% confidence interval for the regression coefficient. This gives an interval for the effect of a £1000 increase in income on travel distance of −0.35 to −0.09 miles. The *P*-value is 0.002, so there is strong evidence against the null hypothesis.

Key Message 14.3: Normality Assumption for Linear Regression

The correct use of linear regression requires the assumption that the errors around the regression line follow a Normal distribution.

Note that the Normality assumption applies to the *errors* around the regression line rather than the original observations. The assumption is only important for small samples.

Extrapolation

Extending the regression line either upwards or downwards in order to make predictions beyond the range of the observed exposure values is known as extrapolation. Making such predictions is best avoided as any linear relationship might not apply outside the observed range, and predicted values may at best be misleading and at worst meaningless.

CORRELATION

Suppose now that we are interested in an overall summary measure of the strength of a relationship between two variables.

> **Key Message 14.4: Correlation**
>
> Correlation shows the strength of association between two continuous variables.

The degree of linear association is generally estimated by Pearson's product moment correlation coefficient (often referred to in articles as Pearson's correlation or just correlation). Correlation values can be between −1 and +1; the extreme values are attained only when points lie exactly on a straight line. If the two variables are independent of each other, the correlation is zero. The proportion of the variation in one variable that is explained by the variation in the other variable is given by the square of the correlation value. A correlation of 0.7 or more is considered relatively strong, as the proportion of the variation explained is close to or in excess of one half. As with regression, it is wise to plot the variables against each other before calculating the correlation coefficient. The plot gives an idea of the likely value of the correlation coefficient, and reveals any non linear trends.

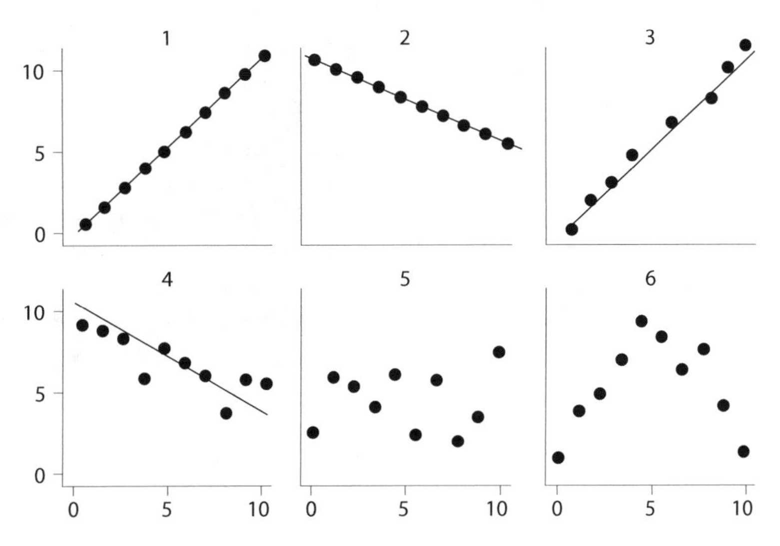

FIGURE 14.2 Scatter diagrams illustrating various types of association.

Figure 14.2 shows six scatter diagrams that illustrate various types of association between two variables. The first depicts perfect positive correlation. Here one variable is totally explained by the other (and hence all the points lie on a straight line). Because the line slopes upwards the correlation is positive. Diagram 2 shows perfect negative correlation. Again the points lie on a straight line, but this time the slope is downwards.

Diagrams 3 and 4 show positive and negative correlation where the relationship is not exact. Most of the points lie away from the fitted lines. Some of the variation in one variable is explained by variation in the other, but there is also some random variation.

Diagram 5 shows completely random variation. Points are scattered all over and there does not appear to be any relation between the two variables. Here the correlation is zero.

Diagram 6 shows data that would need to be treated with caution. The calculated value for the linear correlation is zero, but from the scatter diagram there is evidently a strong association between the two variables that has a non linear form. This illustrates the importance of plotting a scatter diagram first.

Key Message 14.5: Null Hypothesis for Correlation

The appropriate null hypothesis is that in the population from which the sample was taken, the correlation between the two variables is zero.

Example 14.4

In Example 14.1, the null hypothesis is that for the population of young adults the correlation between travel distance and annual income is zero. However, the correlation coefficient between travel distance and annual income is equal to –0.645, indicating a strong negative relationship between the two variables. The 95% confidence interval for the correlation coefficient is from –0.846 to –0.283, indicating that the population value for the correlation is between –0.846 and –0.283 with 95% confidence. The *P*-value of 0.002 shows strong evidence against the null hypothesis.

Key Message 14.6: Normality Assumption for Pearson's Correlation

The correct use of Pearson's correlation requires the assumption that for the population both variables follow a Normal distribution.

The Normality assumption is only required for small samples.

Correlation and Causation

If there are two variables that are associated with each other (giving a fairly high positive correlation, for instance) it is tempting to deduce that one causes the other. Just because an association has been demonstrated does not mean that the two variables can necessarily be linked together in a cause and effect manner. There may be an underlying third variable (sometimes called a confounding variable) that has a genuine relationship with both the variables under consideration. This will give the impression that the two variables being analyzed are linked.

Key Message 14.7: An Important Misunderstanding

Association does not imply causation.

DIFFERENCES AND SIMILARITIES BETWEEN REGRESSION AND CORRELATION COEFFICIENTS

The regression coefficient is the gradient of the regression line and can take any value; the correlation coefficient is the strength of a linear relationship and can take any value between -1 and $+1$ inclusive. Unlike the regression coefficient, the correlation coefficient does not depend on the scale of measurement (e.g., cm or m). Both coefficients are positive if the scatter diagram slope is upwards and negative if the slope is downwards.

> **Key Message 14.8: Link Between Regression and Correlation**
>
> The strength of evidence against the null hypothesis that the population (true) value of the coefficient is 0 (*P*-value) is the same whether the regression coefficient or the correlation coefficient is tested.

AGREEMENT

All the statistical techniques described so far have been based on the assumption that the data being analyzed are reliable. In practice, say in the examination of a tooth for the presence of dental caries, we have two sources of variation. A dentist re-examining the x-ray of a tooth some time later may make a different judgment – this is known as **intra-observer variation**. Also, a colleague may make a different decision about the same tooth, leading to **inter-observer variation**. For both types of variation, the same question can be asked – how well do the two sets of data agree with each other?

> **Key Message 14.9: Agreement and Association**
>
> Agreement is not the same as association. It is possible for the correlation coefficient (a measure of association) to be very high while at the same time the agreement is very low (for instance, if one examiner consistently scores one unit higher than the other).

When relatively few categories are possible, the most obvious measure of agreement between two sets of data is the proportion of cases in which agreement occurs, which is between 0 and 1. However, a substantial amount of agreement can be accounted for by chance alone

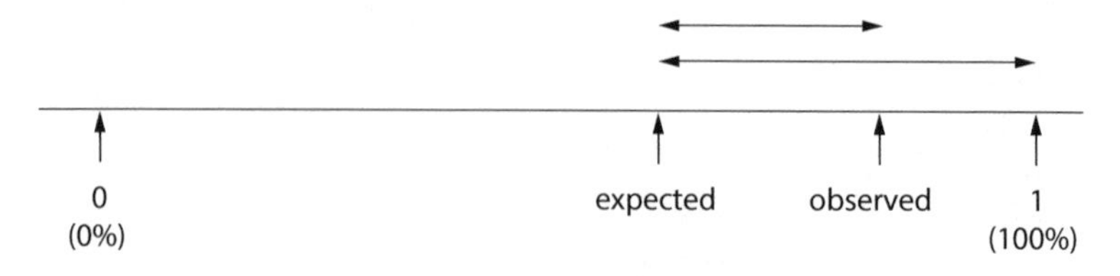

FIGURE 14.3 Chance-corrected agreement.

TABLE 14.1 Decisions of two dentists as to whether patients required treatment or not

	Dentist B		
Dentist A	*Yes*	*No*	*Total*
Yes	40	5	45
No	25	30	55
Total	65	35	100

(consider, for example, two dentists both deciding randomly for each patient in a group whether or not to refer them to a dental hospital).

A measure of agreement that allows for this chance agreement is the proportion of the agreement, over and above that expected by chance, that is actually observed. This approach was proposed by Cohen (1960) and is known as the kappa statistic for chance-corrected agreement. Note that the observed and expected proportions referred to above are often expressed as percentages. In Figure 14.3, kappa is the length of the shorter line as a proportion of the length of the longer line.

Kappa takes the value 1 for perfect agreement, zero for chance agreement and negative values for less than chance agreement. Landis and Koch (1977) suggested that a score of 0.81 or more indicates "almost perfect" agreement, 0.61 to 0.8 indicates "substantial" agreement, and 0.41 to 0.6 "moderate" agreement. Although purely arbitrary, as the authors themselves admitted, these benchmarks are widely used.

Example 14.5

Two dentists inspected 100 patients and rated them as either "requiring treatment" or "not requiring treatment." Table 14.1 shows the decisions of the two dentists.

The observed percentage of agreement is (40 + 30) or 70%. By chance, agreement could be expected on around 50% of the cases. Of the potential agreement remaining (50%), in this study 20% (70–50) is observed (Figure 14.4).

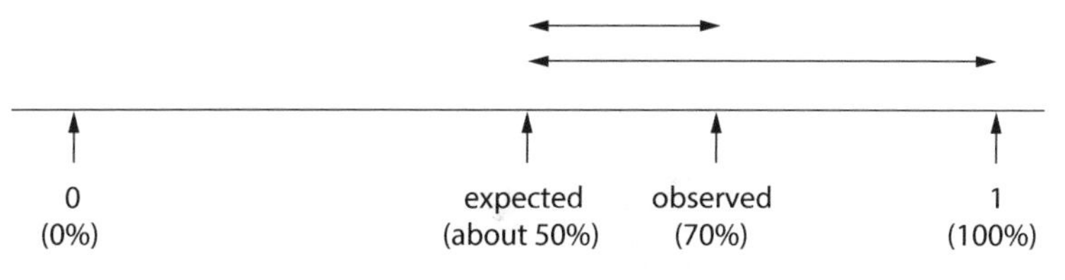

FIGURE 14.4 Chance-corrected agreement for the dentists' decisions in Example 14.5.

This gives a kappa value of around (70–50)/(100–50) or 0.4 (more detailed and accurate calculations are given in the Appendix, see p. 167). On the surface, agreement seems very good but once chance agreement is taken into account the level of agreement is less impressive.

Confidence Intervals for Agreement

Although one can test the null hypothesis that the true value of the kappa statistic is equal to zero, in assessing the level of agreement between trained professionals it is reasonable to assume some agreement beyond that expected by chance. It would be more useful to calculate a 95% confidence interval for kappa, although this involves complex formulae (Fleiss, Leven, and Paik 2003). As with other confidence intervals, these represent the most plausible true values for kappa.

Example 14.6

A study involving 502 young people was conducted into the agreement between the aesthetic component (AC) and dental health component (DHC) of the Index of Orthodontic Treatment Need (Borzabadi-Farahani and Borzabadi-Farahani 2011). The component scores were recorded as treatment needed or not needed. The kappa statistic for diagnostic agreement between the AC and DHC was 0.55 (95% confidence interval from 0.48 to 0.63). We are 95% sure that the population value of kappa was between 0.48 and 0.63. Based on the benchmarks of Landis and Koch (1977) this range of plausible values indicates moderate agreement between the two components.

INTRACLASS CORRELATION

Suppose that two dentists assess the extent of plaque in a series of patients. As part of this assessment, an overall plaque index is calculated by averaging the plaque scores of each tooth surface. In the analysis of their agreement it would be less than ideal to divide these quantitative observations into two categories and calculate the kappa statistic. By doing this, much of the detail in the information would be lost. A means of assessing agreement suitable for quantitative variables is therefore required.

For strong agreement to be present, patients given a high plaque index score by one of the dentists need to have received a high score from the other dentist, with similar relationships existing for the low and intermediate plaque scores. With this in mind, it might be tempting to use Pearson's correlation coefficient to assess the agreement. However, Pearson's correlation is a measure of association and, as noted in Key Message 14.9, agreement and association are different concepts. Two dentists who record plaque index values such that one of the dentists consistently gives a higher score than the other might produce data with a high level of association but not necessarily a high level of agreement. The high value obtained for the Pearson correlation coefficient in this situation may not reflect the truth regarding the level of agreement.

A more suitable measure of agreement is the intraclass correlation coefficient. This has some of the features of Pearson's correlation. For instance, with no link between the two variables (i.e., random variation only) both types of correlation will be equal to 0. The crucial difference between intraclass correlation and Pearson's correlation is that the former is close to 1 only if the level of agreement is high, a more stringent requirement than the strong positive association needed for Pearson's correlation to be close to 1.

A straightforward way of estimating intraclass correlation between two observers involves double entry of the data into adjacent columns in a spreadsheet. Data are entered with the value for Dentist A to the left of that for Dentist B. This process is continued using the same columns but with the values for the two dentists interchanged. The intraclass correlation for the original data is equal to the Pearson correlation of the doubled-up data.

In addition to its use in the assessment of observer agreement, intraclass correlation can be a valuable tool in the study of similarities between twins. If, for instance, dental anxiety scores are obtained from a series of twins, the intraclass correlation between the paired scores provides a measure of similarity for twins in terms of dental anxiety.

Intraclass correlation can be defined for larger groups of individuals, such as the students belonging to a tutorial class within a dental school. If the observations are not independent of each other, as may be the case with the test scores of individual students within a class, the use of basic statistical methods can give misleading results. The (non-zero) value of the intraclass correlation coefficient for the test scores plays an important role in performing the appropriate analyses (Masood, Masood, and Newton 2015).

TEST YOUR UNDERSTANDING

1 What is the most likely value for Pearson's correlation coefficient for the following descriptions of scatter diagrams?

Options:
(a) 0
(b) −0.9
(c) 0.4
(d) 0.8
(e) 1
   (i) Variables seem to be independent of each other.
   (ii) Points lie on a straight upwards-sloping line.
   (iii) Points are close to a straight line sloping downwards.
   (iv) Points are widely scattered around a straight line sloping upwards.
   (v) Points are close to a straight line sloping upwards.

2. Why does an association between two variables not necessarily imply causation? Illustrate with an example from dentistry.
3. Chance-corrected agreement can be close to zero when the observed agreement is high, say 90%. Using an example from dentistry, explain how this could arise.
4. A school-based study was conducted in North Carolina, US into the relationship between untreated decayed primary teeth in kindergarten children (aged around five years) and low household income (Abasaeed, Kranz, and Rozier 2013). The unit of analysis was the school and the main outcome variable was the proportion of kindergarten children in the school with one or more decayed primary teeth (prop dt). The prevalence of low household income was measured by the proportion of the children in the whole school enrolled for free or reduced-price school meals (prop FRSM).
   (i) State an appropriate null hypothesis, at the school level, for the relationship between untreated decayed primary teeth in kindergarten children and low household income.
   (ii) Suggest a possible relationship between these two measures that might be found in practice.

   In an analysis of the 1215 schools involved, the gradient of the regression line of prop dt against prop FRSM was found to be 0.0305 with a 95% confidence interval from 0.001 to 0.0604.

   (iii) Interpret the value 0.0305.
   (iv) What does the 95% confidence interval indicate about the association between these two variables?
   (v) Do these results show a "cause and effect" relationship between low household income and tooth decay in kindergarten children?

CHAPTER 15

Non-Normally Distributed Data

INTRODUCTION

Most of the methods considered so far have been based on the Normal distribution. These may be inapplicable for any of the following reasons:

- Data are continuous but not Normally distributed.
- Data include censored observations, known only to be above or below a particular value.
- Data consist of two independent groups with population variances that are unequal.
- Data are discrete quantitative and so can only take whole number values.
- Data are qualitative, either ordered or unordered.

For discrete quantitative data having many categories, observations may be treated in a similar manner to continuous data. In the qualitative situation, it may be possible to analyze the data as proportions. The emphasis in this chapter will therefore be on methods for continuous data.

TRANSFORMING DATA TO A NORMAL DISTRIBUTION

If the data are not Normally distributed it may be possible to transform the data. Some variables, such as *Lactobacillus* counts, have a positively skewed distribution (Figure 15.1). Most of the counts are of a similar order of magnitude, but a few values are far in excess of the others (there is a long tail in the positive direction). Such distributions can sometimes be transformed into an approximately Normal shape by

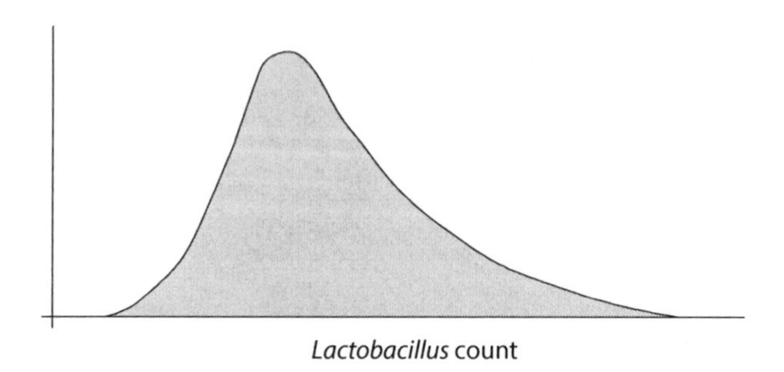

FIGURE 15.1 Original positively skewed data.

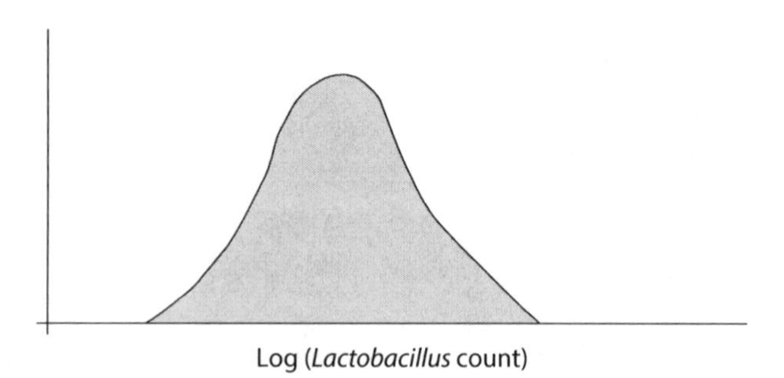

FIGURE 15.2 Positively skewed data following a log transformation.

taking the logarithm of each value (Figure 15.2). For instance, taking logs to base 10 of *Lactobacillus* counts ranging in size from 100 to 1,000,000 leads to transformed values ranging from 2 to 6. The positive skew will thus be reduced if not eliminated.

When comparing two groups, taking logarithms often produces approximately equal variances in populations with different mean values. The methods based on the Normal distribution can then be applied to obtain means and confidence intervals on the logarithmic (log) scale. These confidence intervals need to be "antilogged" if they are required in the original units of measurement.

The log transformation should never be used with negatively skewed distributions (with a long tail towards negative values) as they may contain negative numbers, for which logarithms do not exist. In any case, taking logs will make the data even more negatively skewed. Transformations are inappropriate if some of the observations are not known exactly, as with censored values.

NON-PARAMETRIC METHODS

If the assumption of Normality is not satisfied and/or samples are small, it may be necessary to apply methods that do not depend on the populations having a Normal distribution in order to avoid the possibility of misleading findings. The study of these techniques is a vast area in its own right (Sprent and Smeeton 2007).

> **Key Message 15.1: No Assumed Distribution**
>
> Methods that are not based on an assumed distribution are called non-parametric or distribution-free methods. Remember that it is the methods that are non-parametric, not the data.

The Wilcoxon Two-Sample Test

This test is equivalent to the Mann–Whitney U test, often used in dental journal papers. The assumption that the population distributions are Normal is not required. Hence, the Wilcoxon two-sample test may be appropriate for groups with observations that do not appear to be Normally distributed. The two groups need to be independent of each other.

The null hypothesis is that the two population distributions are the same; if this is not the case the two distributions are assumed to differ only in that their medians are different. (Note that the mean is not generally referred to, as it is an inappropriate average for non-Normal distributions.) Instead of using the data values the two groups are combined and the observations in the pooled data set are ranked.

> **Key Message 15.2: Ranking Data**
>
> The lowest value is given a rank of 1, the next lowest a rank of 2, etc. The highest value has a rank equal to the sample size. If two or more subjects share the same value, the average of the ranks that would have been assigned to those subjects had they differed slightly is given to each subject.

Under the null hypothesis one would expect each group to contain some high-ranking, some low-ranking and some intermediate values. However, if the null hypothesis is not true, high-ranking values will

TABLE 15.1 Overall ranking for the merged male and female groups

Group (gender)	*F*	*F*	*M*	*F*	*M*	*M*	*M*	*M*	*M*
DMFT score	0	2	5	6	7	8	9	10	15
Rank of DMFT score	1	2	3	4	5	6	7	8	9

tend to be found in only one of the groups, with mainly low-ranking values in the other group. Once the ranks have been allocated the sum of the ranks for the smaller group is calculated and compared with the sum expected were the null hypothesis to be true. A *P*-value should also be given.

Example 15.1

The decayed, missed, and filled teeth (DMFT) scores for a group of three females are 0, 2 and 6. For a group of six males the DMFT scores are 5, 7, 8, 9, 10 and 15. The null hypothesis is that the population distribution of DMFT scores is the same for males as for females. The data here suggest that females may have lower DMFT scores on average; that is, less decay. The result of ranking the data is shown in Table 15.1.

The females are the smaller group with ranks that sum to 1+2+4 = 7.

Note that there are no high-rank values in this group. The lowest sum possible is 1+2+3 = 6 and the highest sum possible is 7+8+9 = 24. The sum of ranks is therefore relatively low. The Wilcoxon two-sample test gives a *P*-value of 0.0389, showing some evidence against the null hypothesis. The females appear to have healthier teeth than the males on average.

Key Message 15.3: The Wilcoxon Two-Sample Test and Censored Values

The Wilcoxon two-sample test can sometimes be applied where there are censored observations. For instance, if the largest value in a data set is known only to be above a certain value and/or the lowest value is known only to be less than a certain value, the ranking of the data will remain the same. Whatever their exact values, the lowest value will have a rank of 1 and the highest value will have a rank equal to the sample size.

Kruskal-Wallis Analysis of Variance

This test is a non-parametric alternative to one-way analysis of variance. It operates along the same lines as the Wilcoxon two-sample test and is appropriate for three or more independent groups. The population distributions do not need to satisfy the Normality assumption.

The null hypothesis is that the population distributions are the same; if this is not the case, the distributions are assumed to differ only in that their medians are different. Observations from the groups are pooled and ranked. Under the null hypothesis one would expect each group to contain some high-ranking, some low-ranking and some intermediate values. However, if the null hypothesis is not true, high-ranking values will tend to be found in only some of the groups with mainly low-ranking values in the other groups. The *P*-value given by the test should be reported with the findings.

Spearman's Rank Correlation

This measure of association does not require the assumption that the two population distributions are Normal, as needed for the correct use of Pearson's correlation coefficient. Spearman's correlation is obtained by first ranking the observations for each variable separately and then finding Pearson's correlation for the ranks. As with Pearson's correlation, values lie between −1 and 1, and if the variables are independent of each other, Spearman's correlation takes the value zero.

Unlike Pearson's correlation, the points on the scatter diagram do not need to lie on a straight line for perfect association to occur. If the lines joining adjacent points (moving across horizontally) all have a positive gradient (see Figure 14.2, Diagram 3), Spearman's correlation will be equal to 1; if these lines consistently have a negative gradient, Spearman's correlation will take the value −1.

The appropriate null hypothesis is that in the population from which the sample was taken, Spearman's correlation for the two variables is zero. The hypothesis test produces a *P*-value, and a corresponding 95% confidence interval for the population value of Spearman's correlation can be calculated. If some degree of association is to be expected, results from testing the null hypothesis may add little to what is already known and a 95% confidence interval is much more informative.

TEST YOUR UNDERSTANDING

1 Explain why a simple logarithmic (log) transformation cannot be applied to the data in Example 10.3 showing change in salivary buffering capacity pH.
2 A group of adults aged 18–30 years living in London is to be compared with a similar group living in Edinburgh, using the DMFT score. Name an appropriate statistical test for analyzing the two groups of scores, justifying your choice. In generalizing the results to cities as a whole, what assumptions do we need to make about the samples?
3 Write down a set of observations containing censored values to which the straightforward method of ranking can be applied.
4 Sketch a scatter diagram for which Spearman's rank correlation is around –1 but Pearson's correlation will be closer to zero.

CHAPTER 16

The Choice of Sample Size

INTRODUCTION

It has already been noted that to make the best use of limited resources it is necessary to select a sample of an appropriate size. This decision needs to be made when the study is planned and is based on a sample-size calculation. A statement about the estimated size of the sample required for a study is usually requested by funding organizations and ethical committees when a project proposal is assessed. Sample-size calculation generally involves quite complicated algebra; the interested reader should consult a detailed text on medical statistics, such as Armitage, Berry, and Matthews (2001).

In Chapter 10, hypothesis testing was described in terms of stating a null hypothesis and assessing the strength of evidence against it as judged by the sample collected in the study. Often researchers will have some idea of what the true difference between the groups ought to be. For Example 11.1 this might have been that in the population private practice dentists have on average 10 years' more experience than health service dentists. In a comparison of the dental registration of men and women, it might be that in the population the proportions registered with a dentist are 60% for females and 45% for males. The likely difference is stated explicitly in what is called the alternative hypothesis. This is considered should the null hypothesis appear to be unlikely (Chapter 10).

SOME BASIC CONCEPTS

The sample size required for a study depends on several factors related to the hypothesis testing as follow.

Significance Level

This is the size of the *P*-value for which the strength of evidence against the null hypothesis is sufficiently high for the alternative hypothesis to be considered instead. Traditionally this has been taken as 0.05 since it follows naturally from the favored threshold between acceptance and rejection of the null hypothesis.

Power

This is the probability that the alternative hypothesis is chosen, given that it is actually true. The larger the sample, the smaller the standard error(s) associated with the null hypothesis. Smaller standard errors mean that a sample difference is more likely to appear implausible under the null hypothesis, thus allowing the alternative hypothesis to be chosen. So, a larger sample means higher power. Traditionally this has been taken as 0.8 or occasionally 0.9 (not 0.95, as might be thought). This reflects the fact that a power of 0.95 often leads to unrealistically high sample-size requirements. Also, failure to choose a correct alternative hypothesis has traditionally been regarded as a less serious error than throwing out a perfectly adequate null hypothesis.

One or Two Tails?

In a one-tailed test only differences in one direction are of interest. For instance, in a comparison of male and female registration only differences in proportions for which females have a higher value might be of concern. This approach is generally frowned on, as, were the researchers' initial impressions to be totally wrong, male registration might in fact be higher.

> **Key Message 16.1: The Need for Two-Tailed Tests**
>
> Two-tailed tests are preferable, despite raising the sample-size requirement, because large differences in either direction should not be ignored.

Ratio of the Group Sizes

It can be shown that for any given alternative hypothesis, the number of individuals required is the smallest when the groups are of equal size. If groups of unequal size are planned, this only makes a sizeable difference to the total number required where the ratio of the sizes is large (more than three, say).

Standardized Difference (Used with Means)

For continuous variables it is insufficient just to propose a difference in true means. The power of a test is affected by the size of the true standard deviation of the observations in each group. A large standard deviation implies a lot of overlap between the two groups. The difference in true means is therefore divided by an estimate of the true standard deviation to give the standardized mean difference, also referred to as the effect size of the study. For instance, if the alternative hypothesis states that the true difference in means is 10 and the standard deviation of the observations in the two groups is 20, the standardized mean difference is equal to 0.5.

Key Message 16.2: Effect Size

An effect size is a measure that describes the magnitude of the difference between two groups. If the difference between two group means is of interest, the effect size is equal to the standardized mean difference.

ROUGH APPROXIMATIONS FOR THE SAMPLE SIZE REQUIRED

In the discussion below, the significance level is assumed to be 0.05 and the tests two-tailed.

Comparing Two Proportions

Suppose it is planned that binary (yes/no) data will be analyzed using the test for two proportions described in Chapter 12. From the difference between the proportions as stated in the alternative hypothesis, Table 16.1 gives an upper limit for the number required in each of the two groups. If 0.5 lies between the lower proportion and the higher proportion, Table 16.1 is quite accurate. If both proportions are to one side of 0.5, the actual sample-size requirement is considerably less than the number shown. Table 16.1 can be used to assess the feasibility of a study, but a statistical computing package such as *Stata* (StataCorp 2015) should be used to obtain the exact numbers required.

Example 16.1

Researchers plan to test the null hypothesis that the proportion of 14-year-olds with evidence of dental caries is equal for males and females. They state in an alternative hypothesis that the proportions

TABLE 16.1 Maximum number required in each group to detect a given true difference in proportions – power of 0.8

Difference in proportions	*Number per group*
0.05	1609
0.10	412
0.15	187
0.20	107
0.25	70
0.30	49
0.35	37
0.40	29
0.45	23
0.50	19
0.55	16
0.60	13
0.65	11
0.70	10

are 0.35 for girls and 0.5 for boys. For the alternative hypothesis, the difference in proportions is therefore 0.15. Table 16.1 shows that with a power of 0.8, 187 14-year-olds are required in each group (males, females). This is sufficiently accurate for the purposes of this study; using *Stata* the calculated sample size requirement is 183 individuals per group.

Comparing Two Means

Suppose a study is planned in which the data from two independent groups are to be analyzed as a comparison of two means using the unpaired *t*-test (Chapter 11). If the power is set at 0.8, the rule of 16 (Lehr 1992) gives a rough approximation for the number required in each group of 16 divided by the square of the standardized mean difference. Accurate sample size estimates can be found using *Stata*.

Example 16.2

In Example 11.1, the mean length of experience was 22 years for the private practice dentists and 18 years for the health service dentists, a sample difference of four years. A suitable alternative hypothesis for this study is that for the population the mean difference in length of experience is four years. Given the standard deviations of the two samples (11.57 and 12.42) it would be reasonable to assume a population standard deviation for length of experience in each group of 12 years.

The standardized difference is $4/12 = 1/3$ and so the square of the standardized difference is equal to $1/9$. Using the rule of 16 (power of 0.8), the number of individuals required in planning a study of this type is around 16 divided by $1/9 = 16 \times 9 = 144$ individuals per group or 288 individuals altogether. Using *Stata* the calculated sample-size requirement is 142 individuals per group or 284 in all; in this example the accuracy of Lehr's method is impressive.

TEST YOUR UNDERSTANDING

1. Explain why a study design that allows for a power of 0.5 would be considered unacceptable.
2. Use the rule of 16 to estimate the sample-size requirement where the two means in the alternative hypothesis are 5 and 3, the assumed standard deviation is 2, and a power of 0.8 is required.
3. If a power of 0.9 is required, the sample size requirement can be estimated using the rule of 21. Explain how this rule operates in simple terms. What do the rules of 16 and 21 indicate about the relationship between power and sample size?

CHAPTER 17

Evidence-based Dentistry

INTRODUCTION

Having considered the basic aspects of study design and the application of statistics to observations collected in a dental setting, we now consider an issue that is at the heart of the practice of dentistry. How can the dentist most effectively address the needs and expectations of patients within the constraints of staff availability and in a way that is financially realistic? The application of evidence-based dentistry (EBD) may assist in resolving some of these issues.

THE PURPOSE OF EVIDENCE-BASED DENTISTRY

Evidence-based dentistry can be described as addressing the oral health needs of the patient by making best use of the current scientific evidence in the choice of treatment methods. For dental practitioners primarily engaged in patient care rather than academic research it can be daunting to find the time required to make use of the resources available for acquiring skills in evidence-based dentistry.

The way in which evidence-based dentistry operates bears some resemblance to the "cycle of research" illustrated in Figure 1.1 (population → design → sample → deductions). The EBD process works as follows:

- Decide on a relevant question.
- Identify the best evidence available.
- Appraise the evidence using objective criteria.
- Apply the findings to your patients.
- Evaluate the impact of the modifications on your patient care.

Key Message 17.1: The Evidence Base Should Be Updated Regularly

The EBD process should be repeated regularly so that new findings are added to the knowledge base.

SYSTEMATIC REVIEWS

Sources of Information

Once a relevant and answerable question has been chosen, a comprehensive review of the sources of information available on the topic should be carried out. In particular, articles published in refereed dental and medical journals should be identified, along with other peer-reviewed material. Most of these documents can be identified and obtained via comprehensive databases accessible through the Internet. Each online database has its own sophisticated search facility so that documents can be identified through the use of keywords, author names, dates of publication, etc. Important sources, listed alphabetically, include the following.

- Cochrane Library.
  A group of databases primarily for medicine and other health-care specialties provided by the Cochrane Collaboration. At its core is the collection of Cochrane Reviews on specific topics, e.g., water fluoridation for the prevention of dental caries (Iheozor-Ejiofor et al. 2015).
- EMBASE
  Its main focus is on medicine, covering publications from 1947.
- MEDLINE (Medical Literature Analysis and Retrieval System Online)
  Arguably the most well-known database, it covers publications in biomedicine and health from 1950.
- Ovid
  This database provides access to academic journals and other online documents, mainly in health sciences.
- PsychInfo
  This database covers (mainly) publications in psychology from 1967.
- PubMed
  This is a search engine primarily designed for accessing MEDLINE.

- SciELO
  Designed for research conducted in developing countries. Useful for identifying non-English literature, especially work published in Spanish and Portuguese.
- ScienceDirect
  This database operates as a platform for access to academic journals and e-books. It covers physical sciences, engineering, life sciences, health sciences, social sciences, and humanities from 1997.
- WEB OF SCIENCE
  This citation indexing service contains details of articles in science, social science, arts, and humanities published since 1900.

Additional sources of potentially useful papers include:

- "Grey" literature (e.g., government publications, health authority internal reports). Although these documents are generally given public access, if not online they can be difficult to locate.
- Searching journals by hand.
- Checking the cited references in the papers identified in the initial searches.
- Direct contact with researchers working in the fields of interest.

Key Message 17.2: Using Multiple Databases

It is unlikely that one database alone will identify all of the publications of interest.

Example 17.1

Hayden et al. (2013) published a systematic review on obesity and dental caries in children. A literature search was carried out using the databases EMBASE, MEDLINE, ScienceDirect, Ovid and PsychInfo. The search was restricted to studies published in English between 1980 and 2010. The keywords used in the searches were: obes* [i.e., any word starting with obes], child*, pediatric, weight, overweight, BMI, dental caries, primary dentition, dft, dmft, dmfs, dfs.

Hierarchy of Research

Since research investigations are conducted using a range of study designs and given that some adhere to the agreed protocol more closely than others, it is useful to be able to rate a study according to

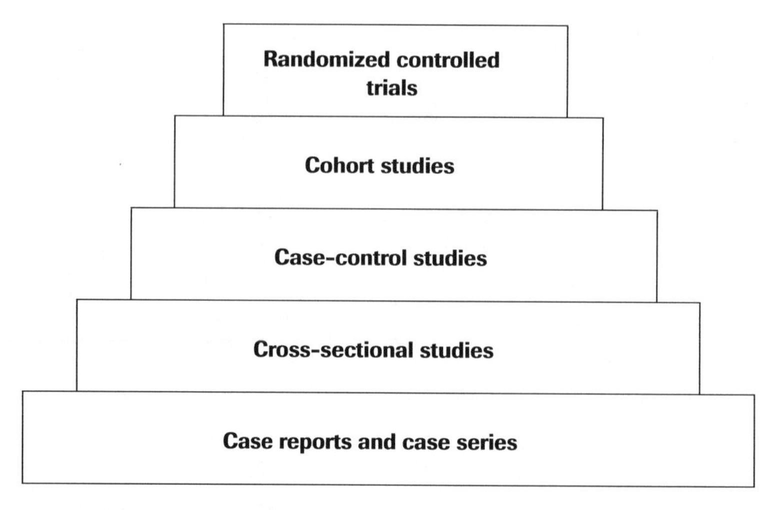

FIGURE 17.1 Levels of evidence in the context of study design.

its level of evidence and the quality of its findings. Although there is no universally adopted convention in terms of defining specific levels of evidence, it is generally accepted that results from an overall analysis of objectively selected randomized controlled trials are of greatest value, while anecdotal information and expert opinion contribute the least. A simple representation of the main components of this hierarchy of research is shown in Figure 17.1.

Research Quality

Each study should be appraised in terms of any actual or potential flaws in its design and conduct. If a study has significant weaknesses (e.g., important records are missed in a case-control study, blinding that could have been applied in a randomized controlled trial is overlooked), its sub-optimal quality will reduce its contribution to the overall body of knowledge.

> **Key Message 17.3: Poor-Quality Research**
>
> Results from a poorly conducted randomized controlled trial may be of no more value than those from a less sophisticated but well-conducted investigation.

Publications in Languages Other Than English

Almost all dental research papers are written in English. However, other languages are in use. Some articles published in journals based in South America are available only in Spanish or Portuguese; most of these have an English Language abstract. Articles written in languages other than English may be worth considering in a systematic review, particularly if multilingual colleagues are willing to assist. The quality of these studies tends to be lower compared to those published in international journals as indicated below.

Example 17.2
Moraga (2014) investigated the levels of evidence for research published in Chilean dental journals during 2012. Of the 120 papers published, just three reported on a randomized controlled trial and two on a cohort study. Four of these high-quality research papers were in Spanish but all had an English abstract.

META-ANALYSIS

Once a systematic review has been carried out, it is possible to produce a quantitative summary of the evidence obtained from the studies by performing a meta-analysis. Why might we wish to do this?

Small studies on their own may lack the statistical power required to demonstrate differences between the groups of interest, but by combining the findings from similar studies it may be possible to provide strong evidence for differences given the much larger combined sample. Another benefit of comparing a number of studies is that each study may be influenced by factors such as its location; a meta-analysis can highlight these differences. This section gives a general overview of how a meta-analysis is performed rather than an account of the specific details, which can be quite technical from a statistical point of view.

A meta-analysis is only of value if it is based on a comprehensive systematic review of relevant publications. Once this review has been obtained it is necessary to perform quality assessments on the individual papers in order to identify those suitable for inclusion in the meta-analysis. Adding in poor-quality papers may lead to bias in the overall findings, so it is important that the same objective criteria are applied consistently across all of the publications under consideration.

Meta-analyses are based on a variable of interest (e.g., level of dental caries) and a specific measure (e.g., mean). For each study included, the effect size between the groups under comparison is calculated along with the 95% confidence interval for the difference between the groups. This information, along with the sample sizes for each study, provides the basic building blocks for the meta-analysis. Performing the meta-analysis provides a 95% confidence interval for the combined data. With some types of design, defining the effect size can be quite complex, but for a comparison of two group means, the effect size is the standardized mean difference (Chapter 16).

Key Message 17.4: Sensitivity Analysis

It is good practice to perform a sensitivity analysis in order to ascertain the effect of including or excluding studies of uncertain quality. This explores the degree to which the findings from the meta-analysis are influenced by material for which it is difficult to make a decision on whether or not it should be included.

Example 17.3

The paper on obesity and dental caries in children discussed in Example 17.1 (Hayden et al. 2013) reported several meta-analyses of the papers identified by the systematic review. Eight papers were included in a meta-analysis of dental caries in primary dentition. Two of the studies gave evidence for a greater level of dental caries in the obese group relative to children with a normal Body Mass Index. A further study demonstrated a lower level of dental caries in the obese group and the remaining five studies produced no strong evidence for a difference in either direction. The combined data indicated a slight disadvantage for obese children but no strong evidence for an overall effect.

The results reported above appear to be contradictory. However, the studies with equivocal findings were conducted in countries with an established industrial sector. The two investigations in which obese children were at a disadvantage took place in newly industrialized countries where a transition from a traditional diet to a Western (high sugar) diet is taking place and obesity may be more closely associated with sugar consumption.

IMPLEMENTATION AND EVALUATION

Recommendations for professional dental practice obtained from an evidence-based process will only be effective if applied by dentists to the treatment of their own patients. Changes that need to be implemented may depend on the demographic profile of the patients (age, gender, ethnicity, etc.), the type of care involved (e.g., routine inspection, restorative care, aesthetics), and the geographical location of the practice. For instance, the findings from Example 17.3 suggest that the provision of dietary advice to children and their parents should be given higher priority if the dentist is based in a newly industrialized country.

Following the implementation of changes in practice it is important that their impact is evaluated by a clinical audit (Johnson and Quinn 2011). This systematic critical analysis of the quality of dental care is best performed once the changes have been in place for an adequate period of time. The audit should highlight the benefits and any difficulties that have arisen. A satisfactory evaluation will justify the retention of the modifications subject to routine re-evaluation.

Example 17.4

In a study of the implementation of evidence-based dentistry conducted in six European countries (Yamalik et al. 2015) an overwhelming proportion (89%) of the participating dentists agreed that evidence-based dentistry is beneficial, but only around one-third (32%) reported that they practiced EBD. Crucially, 60% believed that dentists experience difficulties in implementing EBD, with younger dentists in particular citing lack of time as an issue.

Although agreement on the value of evidence-based dentistry is growing within the dental profession, less certain is the jump from evaluation to implementation. The challenge ahead is the creation of a shift from minimum reasonable standards of care to recommended best practice (Rattan, Chambers, and Wakeley 2002) through the application of evidence-based dentistry.

TEST YOUR UNDERSTANDING

1 Give reasons as to why a journal article might not be identified in a database search.

2 Gomes et al. (2011) analyzed the levels of evidence of the studies published in the journal *Stomatos* between 1995 and 2009. Locate and read this open access paper. Comment on their findings.

3 In the investigation of the literature on dental caries in children conducted by Hayden et al. (2013), the studies listed for the meta-analysis of primary teeth were not exactly the same as those listed for the meta-analysis of permanent teeth, although some of the studies did appear on both lists. What does this indicate about the studies identified?

CHAPTER 18

Statistical Refereeing

INTRODUCTION

Once a piece of research has been completed it is generally expected that the findings will be communicated through one or more academic papers. Indeed, it was one of the stated objectives of the general dental practice research network described in Example 1.1 (Kay, Ward, and Locker 2003). High-quality undergraduate student projects can also lead to publication (Lee et al. 2015). Tutors should therefore encourage their students to view this as a target should the project work be well conducted and interesting.

Not only is it a satisfying experience to have one's paper accepted for publication, it is becoming essential as higher education establishments strive to compete in terms of their research and publication record. For undergraduates, one or more publications at this early stage can considerably enhance their curriculum vitae.

Key Message 18.1: Importance of Publishing in Refereed Journals

For publications to be seen as credible they need to appear in refereed journals, for which papers are assessed by reviewers (often known as referees) and modified in the light of their reports before acceptance.

Building up the skills needed to write effectively is a lifelong process; there is always so much more to learn. The comprehensive and readable book by Day and Gastel (2016) gives much valuable advice on how to write the various sections of a scientific paper. Furthermore, it gives a detailed explanation of the publication process, looking at the roles of authors, referees, editors, and publishers. The purpose of this chapter, however, is to focus on the contribution of the statistical referee. Although today almost all dental journals have a review process along the lines described, some of my specific comments may be influenced by my own experience as statistical adviser for dental research studies, co-author of papers submitted to dental journals, and as a referee.

THE PURPOSE AND CHOICE OF STATISTICAL REFEREES

The main role of the statistical referee is to provide a critical assessment of the statistical aspects of a paper submitted for possible publication. This will supplement the reports obtained from one or more dentally qualified reviewers who are expert in the clinical content of the paper. The editor uses these reports to obtain an overall impression of the quality of the paper and decide on whether it should be accepted, modified for further review, or rejected. Statistical referees can be involved throughout the whole of this process, although some journals send out to statisticians only those papers judged to be of reasonable clinical content.

Reports provided by referees (statistical and dental) often have a particular structure specific to that journal. Reviewers may be asked to complete an initial tick-box questionnaire on their overall impression of each of the main sections of the paper (abstract, introduction, methods, results, etc.). All referees provide a detailed report for the authors. I usually commence with a positive remark, perhaps about the context of the study. The main purpose of this report, however, is to highlight the paper's weaknesses, making reference to the text, comments often being segregated into major and minor points. Suggestions on how these weaknesses might be remedied are also provided, with references to appropriate texts or articles if necessary. Normally a referee does not indicate an editorial recommendation in the report for the authors but instead includes this in a set of confidential comments for the editor.

The issue of anonymity is hotly debated. Most journals provide anonymous referee reports. In addition, in recent years, some journals have not disclosed the names of the authors to those who referee their paper. The intention behind this change is to narrow the perceived gap between high-profile authors, whose work is allegedly sought after by editors and readily accepted, and their less experienced colleagues. However, it is claimed by those who defend the traditional position that referees are often able to deduce authorship from the list of references and remarks made within the paper.

Key Message 18.2: Overlap of Content in Statistical and Clinical Reviews

Although statistical referees focus on the statistical issues within a paper and the clinical referees on the clinical aspects, there might be overlap in their reports. A statistician might have experience of dental issues from working on relevant research projects, and some dentists have a good understanding of basic statistics.

In a paper on dental public health in the United Kingdom, I would query a child dental registration rate of 6%, thinking that a zero might have been omitted. Conversely, a dental referee might well remark on the statement "$P > 0.05$, statistically significant," the inequality sign being incorrect. Hence, it is perfectly possible that more than one referee might comment on a particular error.

The issue of the limits of expertise can be a sensitive one, and I know of more than one statistician who has resigned from refereeing for a particular journal because of being asked to review a paper "from a statistical point of view." Some statisticians prefer to decide on their own boundaries; dealing with statistical referees can require an editor to show a good measure of tact!

Those selected as statistical referees usually have a first degree in either mathematics or statistics and in addition either a taught postgraduate qualification or a research degree based around medical statistics. Ideally, statisticians with experience of involvement in dental research are sought, but a study in Britain and Ireland has shown that a significant amount of undergraduate dental statistics teaching is conducted by dentally qualified staff, thus it is more than likely that statisticians with a research background in dentistry are scarce (Smeeton 2002). Hence, in the United Kingdom at least, medical statisticians form the main supply of statistical referees for dental journals.

In general, editors use a selection of statistical referees, sending each a few papers to review each year. Suitable referees can be difficult to find at short notice so to ensure that a statistician is readily available, a journal might appoint a statistical editor, who takes overall responsibility for the quantitative issues raised by the papers submitted. Referees are frequently appointed through acquaintance with the editor, perhaps through working in the same dental school, or by the recommendation of a serving statistical referee. A statistician who co-authors a paper that is accepted for publication in a dental journal may well be asked to consider acting as a reviewer by the journal's editor. Statisticians occasionally offer their services directly to editors. Although some journals pay reviewers for their reports, many statistical referees perform their work on a purely voluntary basis. A few of the journals with an online submissions and review system allow authors to suggest potential referees and list those that they would prefer not to be approached. Editors are not obliged to contact referees selected by authors.

CONFLICTS OF INTEREST

Referees should be impartial and comment objectively on all papers that they review. Occasionally this is not possible, as one or more of the authors is well known to the referee (this is one argument that could be made for blind refereeing). There may be a temptation for the referee to produce a more favorable report than would otherwise be written. In such a situation it is proper for the individual to contact the editor requesting that an alternative referee be approached. Referees also need to inform the editor if they have already reviewed the paper for another journal. Other conflicts of interest occasionally arise; for example, a referee may have a financial interest in the pharmaceutical company that has funded the research described in the paper to be reviewed. In all cases of doubt the prudent course of action is for the referee to contact the journal editor.

> **Key Message 18.3: Conflicts of Interest – Authors**
>
> Some journals require authors to state any conflicts of interest involved in their research; even if this is not requested, it is good practice for authors to mention any conflicts of interest to the editor on initial submission or indicate that there are no such difficulties.

Authors should not submit a paper to more than one journal at a time. If one of the journals chooses to publish the paper, the submission may be withdrawn from the other journal(s), possibly when their referees have already spent time assessing it. Some journals request authors to provide reviews obtained from previous submissions of the manuscript to other journals and indicate how the paper has been revised to take these comments into account.

THE INVOLVEMENT OF STATISTICIANS IN DENTAL RESEARCH

The discussion so far may have given the impression that statisticians have primarily a negative role in the preparation of papers. However, they can make an important contribution before a paper is submitted. If a dental research team does not include a qualified statistician, statistical advice should be sought as soon as the nature of the project has been decided and definitely before the detailed design of the study has been chosen. For investigators applying for financial assistance from grant-awarding bodies, evidence of such advice being given and taken is normally expected on the funding application forms. Many funding bodies have statisticians who assess applications with a particular focus on the design and analysis of the proposed study. In addition, ethical committees frequently require evidence that statistical advice has been applied in drawing up the study proposal. In particular, a statement about a sample-size calculation should be given, which usually needs a statistician's help. A statistician can also assist in the choice of study design including sampling techniques and methods of randomization for clinical trials.

Most statisticians are familiar with the heart-sink experience of being approached only after the data have been collected, leaving the researchers unsure about how to proceed. Although it is better to involve a statistician at this late stage than not at all, if a study is badly designed it can be irredeemably flawed. It may be impossible to rectify such a study purely by the use of statistical techniques, however sophisticated. An even worse situation is one in which a researcher approaches a statistician only on receiving a negative statistical referee's report.

If the involvement of a statistician in a study is likely to be substantial, it is appropriate to consider the statistician as a collaborator and co-author on any papers that are produced. (Most established statisticians see little personal value in being included in a list of acknowledgements and would only be happy with this if their contribution to a study has been small.) This gives the investigators ready access to statistical advice throughout the study, supervision of the analysis, and assistance in the preparation of any articles for possible publication. A statistical collaborator is in a position to defend any negative comments on the statistical aspects of a paper made by the referees.

Where undergraduate students working together on a research project consider publication, it is advisable and respectful to approach the supervisor initially. The project supervisor should be able to make a judgment about the project's suitability and which journals, if any, could be approached. Supervisors may need to request assistance from statistical colleagues. Some institutions offer statistical teaching programs to registered research students. This can involve lectures, seminars, practical computing sessions, and assessment.

COMMON PROBLEMS OF A STATISTICAL NATURE

Key Message 18.4: Do Not Expect Referees to Rewrite Your Paper for You

A paper should not be submitted until all the imperfections about which the authors are aware have been corrected. Reducing the number of probable modifications required by the referees makes outright rejection less likely and speeds up the process between initial submission and final acceptance.

A paper submitted to a dental journal will rarely be rejected because of its statistical aspects alone. However, where the paper overall is seen as borderline, poor study design, data presentation, or statistical analysis can be deciding factors between a request for revision or rejection. It is therefore worthwhile to pay attention to these aspects, checking the paper with a statistician before submission. This section is intended to give an indication of the more common problems encountered by a statistical referee. To keep things simple, the examples will mainly be drawn from issues already discussed in this text. These are not intended to be comprehensive, but they do show that involving a statistician can make things much smoother in the refereeing process. Altman et al. (2000) give detailed advice on preparing manuscripts.

Table 18.1 shows some common deficiencies with the "Introduction" and "Methods." It is possible that some of these would also be commented on by a dental referee. Issues of background and presentation can be corrected without too much difficulty, but problems with poor study design can be beyond correction once the investigation has been completed.

TABLE 18.1 Some common problems with the Introduction and Methods

Problem	*Effect*	*Corrective action*
Key references to previous work overlooked	Reader has incomplete picture of current knowledge	Authors to add references given by the referees and perform further literature searches
No sample-size calculation	Unclear as to whether authors planned the sample size in advance	Add results of calculation or indicate what size of difference might have been detected by the study
Sampling excludes patients of a particular ethnic group	Findings cannot be generalized to the whole population	Not usually possible to rectify afterwards. Results should be presented in the limited context of the patients represented in the sample
Age recorded in 10-year intervals	Limited information about age distribution	Impossible to rectify unless exact age can be obtained from dental records or by asking participants again
In a clinical trial, patients allocated to groups by clinician's discretion	Likelihood of underlying differences between groups on patient characteristics	Impossible to adjust to randomized sampling afterwards (NB: paper likely to be rejected)

Table 18.2 indicates potential deficiencies in the "Results," "Discussion," and "Conclusions." Aspects of presentation and analysis are usually possible to modify, although changes in statistical methods used can involve a substantial amount of effort. The findings of the study might change; the conclusions will then need to be reconsidered.

Statistical referees are only human and are therefore capable of omitting to point out a particular deficiency or giving unwarranted emphasis to a problem with the paper. It is wise to ask a statistician to read through the statistical (and other) comments made by the referees. A statistician should be able to assist in arguing the statistical points in a rebuttal should an appeal against a rejection decision be made (see next section).

In order to assist authors in the statistical aspects of manuscript preparation, some journals incorporate detailed advice in any guidelines that they produce for authors. For instance, the *British Dental Journal* encourages the presentation of exact P-values in preference to statements such as "$P > 0.05$".

TABLE 18.2 Some common problems with the Results, Discussion, and Conclusions

Problem	*Effect*	*Corrective action*
Percentages in tables given without frequencies	Size of sample on which tables were based is unclear	Add appropriate numbers to tables
Three-dimensional pie charts used for categorical data	Sizes of the various slices are distorted	Change to two-dimensional pie charts or bar charts
Paired data analyzed as two independent groups	Incorrect confidence intervals and *P*-values, hence misleading conclusions	Perform an appropriate paired analysis
A test assuming a Normal population (e.g., *t*-test) is applied to skewed data	Confidence intervals and *P*-values misleading as Normal assumptions are invalid	Analysis to be carried out with an appropriate non-parametric test (e.g., Wilcoxon two-sample test)
Treatment groups analyzed as found at the end of the study	Bias introduced as those who change treatments or drop out are not typical	Intention to treat analysis based on the original treatment groups should be undertaken
Remarks such as "$P > 0.05$, significant"	Statement is nonsense, confusing the reader	Give exact *P*-value and indicate strength of evidence against the null hypothesis
Findings of other researchers misinterpreted	Misleading impression of what the authors are adding to current knowledge	Discussion should be rewritten accurately
Inappropriate conclusions, given the results of the study	Reader misled or confused	Conclusions should be reconsidered

REPORTS AND DECISIONS

Once an editor has received a paper, it is normally sent out to referees chosen by the editor on the basis of the paper's contents. It is rare for an editor to accept a paper for publication immediately. A paper can be returned to the authors without assessment if its theme is not within the subject areas covered by the journal. For instance, a paper on an aspect of dental public health will probably not be seen by referees if it is sent to a journal for oral surgery. The editor might suggest more suitable journals in his or her letter of reply. Papers may also face immediate rejection if they replicate work that has recently been published elsewhere, if the research described is obviously flawed, or if the paper is of a poor general standard. This outcome is more likely with high-circulation journals, which receive far more articles than they can possibly publish. The popularity of these journals is due to their "impact factor," a widely published score that is calculated for each journal on the basis of its circulation and degree of citation of its articles.

Once the initial screening has taken place, the first stage of the refereeing process is set in motion. In due course, the referees' reports are received by the editor, and based on the comments, an editorial decision is made. The most likely outcomes are immediate acceptance (this is rare), acceptance subject to minor amendments, reconsideration subject to major revision, or rejection. Authors submitting a revised manuscript are sometimes asked to respond to the referees' comments on a point-by-point basis in a separate document. This process is repeated until the editor is left with making a final decision of either publication or rejection. The final decision is usually based on the degree of amendment suggested by the referees and how closely the authors have followed their advice. The editors may accept a revised paper without all the referees' comments being acted upon, but authors need to give a reasonable explanation regarding those points not taken up.

Referees are normally expected to provide reports within a reasonable period of time. In practice, depending on the expectations and reminders of the editor, this can vary from one week to several months. Online submission and review have helped expedite the process. From my experience, this has significantly reduced the time required by a referee to produce and submit a detailed report. If authors have not received reports by two or three months, it is not unreasonable for them to ask the editor for an update on their paper's progress in the review process. If this request is made politely, it should not prejudice the final decision on the paper.

Appeals against editorial decisions are generally futile where immediate rejection is concerned. However, where a paper has been rejected on the basis of referees' reports an appeal might be worthwhile if at least one of the reports is positive. If this is the authors' decision, the editor should be contacted. Reconsideration of a paper, if initiated, can involve new referees.

Once a paper has been accepted for publication it undergoes an editing and proofreading process by copyeditors and the authors. It is extremely rare for the offer of publication to be withdrawn by the editor at this stage. That would probably only happen in practice should plagiarism or fraudulent presentation of findings be involved. Such conduct is, of course, reprehensible, and the authors are then required to withdraw their paper immediately.

Key Message 18.5: Online Journals

In order to enable prompt publication and encourage a wide readership, some journals are totally online and have open access to all. The costs involved are covered by a publication charge paid by the authors once the article has been accepted. This fee is not an alternative to refereeing but is an additional consideration. The charge is typically reduced for authors based in low-income countries.

Just because a paper is published does not necessarily mean that it is correct or that it reflects commonly held views. *The Lancet* has a Department of Error section designed for the correction of factual statements. The *British Medical Journal* has a rapid response facility that can be accessed electronically. Following the publication of a *BMJ* paper, readers are able to submit comments on the article; this feedback is published as it stands unless it contains obvious inaccuracies or is of an offensive nature. Many other journals publish letters of response from readers to which the authors of the original paper may give a published reply.

The foregoing description has possibly made the task of publishing in a scientific dental journal seem daunting. My intention is not to deter prospective authors but rather to indicate some of the important considerations with a view to increasing the likelihood of success. So, if you have conducted your research well and have the material for an interesting and convincing paper, I would encourage you to take the plunge!

Appendix

7: THE NORMAL DISTRIBUTION

Once data have been collected, an idea will be needed of the middle value or average and the amount of variation around this average or spread: Are the data generally close to the average or widely spread out?

(Arithmetic) Mean

The arithmetic mean is an average found by adding up all the values and dividing by the number of observations. For example, if there are three observations of 3, 4 and 8, the mean is $\frac{3+4+8}{3} = \frac{15}{3}$ or 5. Mean values are substantially influenced by unusual values (outliers) so it is most suitable for distributions that are roughly symmetrical.

Histograms

The histogram is an appropriate method for depicting continuous data. Values are grouped into intervals, generally of equal size. These

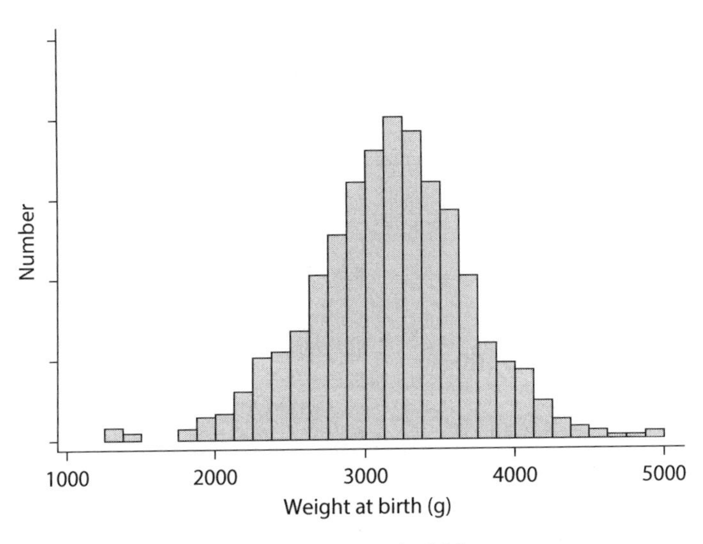

FIGURE A1 A symmetrical histogram.

intervals are then represented by bars with (if intervals have equal width) heights proportional to the frequency of observations contained within them (Figure A1 shows a histogram that is broadly symmetrical).

The Standard Deviation

This is a measure of variability or spread. Each value of the variable will differ from the mean by a certain amount; if the differences tend to be wide, the spread is large. To calculate the standard deviation, take each of these differences and square it; the sum of these squared values is then divided by (n−1), where n indicates the size of the sample. The standard deviation is the square root of this quantity. It is widely used because it is in the same units as the original observations. The standard deviation can be calculated by making use of the s_{n-1} key on most calculators.

Skewed Distributions

Many distributions that are not symmetrical nevertheless have only one peak. These can be divided into those that are positively skewed, with a long tail towards positive values (Figure A2) and those that are negatively skewed, with a long tail towards negative values (Figure A3).

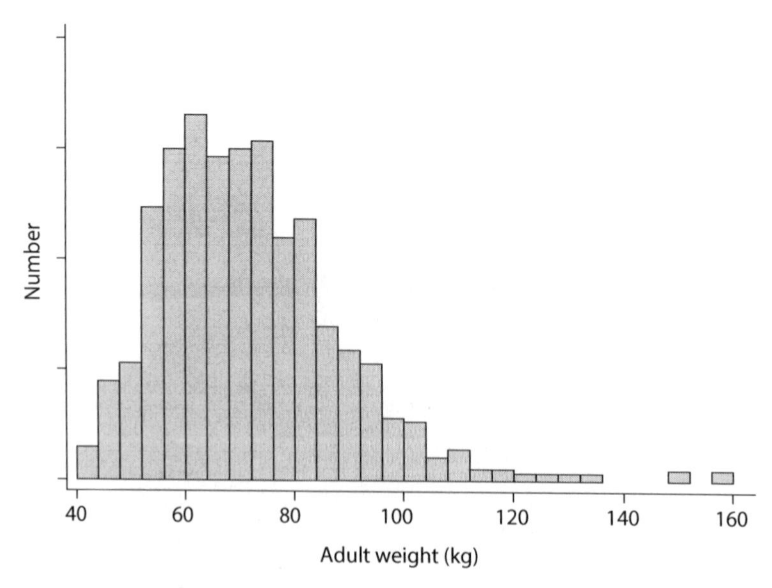

FIGURE A2 A positively skewed histogram.

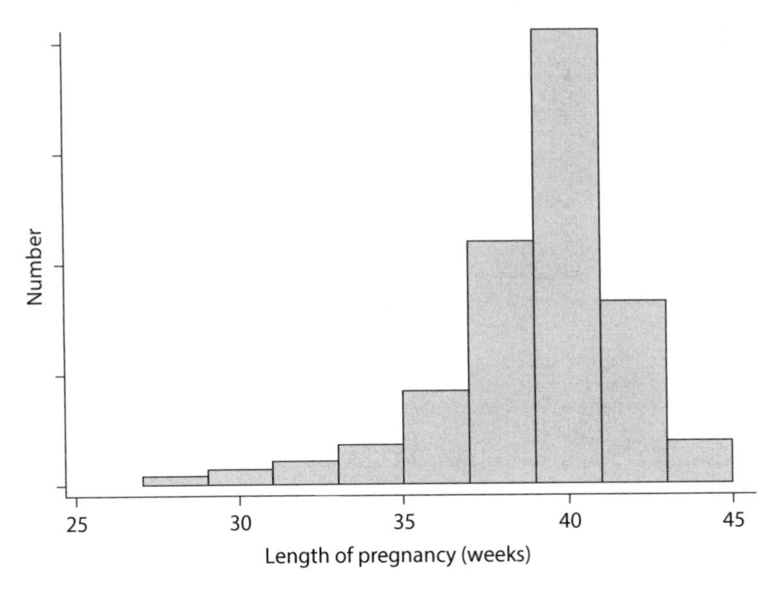

FIGURE A3 A negatively skewed histogram.

9: SAMPLING VARIATION

The Central Limit Theorem

If large samples (usually of size greater than 60) of independent observations are taken from a population having any distribution, as the samples continue to be drawn:

- The sample means will have an approximately Normal distribution.
- The mean of the sample means will be approximately the same as the true population mean.
- The standard deviation of the sample means (standard error or se) can be calculated by dividing the population standard deviation (sd) by the square root of the sample size (n), where n is the number in each sample.

Calculating a 95% Confidence Interval

From Chapter 7, for a Normal distribution 95% of values lie within 1.96 standard deviations of the mean. Sample means are Normally distributed around the population mean, with a standard deviation given by the standard error (se). So 95% of all possible samples will have a mean within 1.96 standard errors of the population mean, i.e., between (population mean – 1.96 × se) and (population mean + 1.96 × se).

However, the sample mean is known, and information is required about the population mean.

If sample mean = population mean – 1.96 × se

then population mean = sample mean + 1.96 × se

Similarly

If sample mean = population mean + 1.96 × se

then population mean = sample mean – 1.96 × se

So the above statements can be reversed, in other words:

We are 95% confident that the true population mean will lie in the range from sample mean – (1.96 × se) to sample mean + (1.96 × se).

This range is called a 95% confidence interval.

Standard Error for a Proportion

As with the sample mean, the standard error is related to the square root of the sample size and is smaller for larger samples. In fact, the standard error of p is estimated by:

$$se = \sqrt{\frac{p(1-p)}{n}}$$

(the square root of "the proportion with the characteristic multiplied by the proportion without the characteristic divided by the sample size").

12: DEALING WITH PROPORTIONS AND CATEGORICAL DATA

95% Confidence Interval for the Population Difference in Proportions

Consider, for example, the effect of fluoridation of water on the incidence of dental caries in adolescents (see Examples 12.1, 12.2, pp. 98 and 99).

Let

n_1 = number of adolescents from the non-fluoridated area
n_2 = number of adolescents from the fluoridated area
p_1 = sample proportion with caries from the non-fluoridated area
p_2 = sample proportion with caries from the fluoridated area

The standard error for the difference between two proportions is given by:

$$\text{Standard error of } (p_1 - p_2) = \sqrt{\frac{p_1(1-p_1)}{n_1} + \frac{p_2(1-p_2)}{n_2}}$$

For Example 12.2

$p_1 = 30/100 = 0.3$ $p_2 = 24/120 = 0.2$

$n_1 = 100$ $n_2 = 120$

$$\text{Standard error of difference} = \sqrt{\frac{0.3(1-0.3)}{100} + \frac{0.2(1-0.2)}{120}}$$

$$= 0.0586$$

Hypothesis Test: The Standard Error for the Difference Between Two Proportions

Let the number with the characteristic of interest be r_1 in the first sample and r_2 in the second sample. If the null hypothesis is true, the best estimate of the overall proportion is p, where:

$$p = \frac{(r_1 + r_2)}{(n_1 + n_2)}$$

$$\text{standard error of } (p_1 - p_2) = \sqrt{p(1-p)\left(\frac{1}{n_1} + \frac{1}{n_2}\right)}$$

$$z = \frac{p_1 - p_2}{se(p_1 - p_2)}$$

In Example 12.3, the null hypothesis is that the population proportion of adolescents with caries is the same in the fluoridated and non-fluoridated areas (see p. 100). The estimate of the overall proportion is given by:

$$p = (30 + 24)/(100 + 120) = 0.2455$$

$$\text{Standard error of } (p_1 - p_2) = \sqrt{0.2455(1-0.2455)\left(\frac{1}{100} + \frac{1}{120}\right)}$$

$$= 0.0583$$

TABLE A.1 Distribution of dental caries in the adolescent samples

	Non-fluoridated	*Fluoridated*	*Total*
Caries	30	24	$r_1 = 54$
No caries	70	96	$r_2 = 166$
Total	$n_1 = 100$	$n_2 = 120$	$N = 220$

The Chi-Squared Test

In Example 12.4 (see p. 101):

Let

n_1 = number of adolescents from the non-fluoridated area
n_2 = number of adolescents from the fluoridated area
r_1 = number of adolescents with caries
r_2 = number of adolescents without caries
N = total number of adolescents (Table A.1)

The null hypothesis is that the population proportion of adolescents with caries is equal in the fluoridated and non-fluoridated areas. If this is true, the distribution of caries should be the same in the two populations. For example, overall a proportion $\frac{r_1}{N}$ of adolescents had caries. So one would expect $n_1 \times \frac{r_1}{N}$ of the adolescents from the non-fluoridated area to have caries.

In this way a table of expected values can be constructed (Table A.2).

For these data the expected values are as shown in Table A.3.

Now assess how much the observed values (O) differ from those expected (E):

For each cell in the table, calculate $\frac{(O-E)^2}{E}$, then add these numbers together to obtain the chi-squared statistic (χ^2).

TABLE A.2 Expected distribution of dental caries in adolescent samples (general case)

	Non-fluoridated	*Fluoridated*	*Total*
Caries	$n_1 \times \frac{r_1}{N}$	$n_2 \times \frac{r_1}{N}$	r_1
No caries	$n_1 \times \frac{r_2}{N}$	$n_2 \times \frac{r_2}{N}$	r_2
Total	n_1	n_2	N

TABLE A.3 Expected distribution of dental caries for the data from Example 12.1

	Non-fluoridated	*Fluoridated*	*Total*
Caries	$100 \times (54/220) = 24.545$	$120 \times (54/220) = 29.455$	$r_1 = 54$
No caries	$100 \times (166/220) = 75.455$	$120 \times (166/220) = 90.545$	$r_2 = 166$
Total	$n_1 = 100$	$n_2 = 120$	$N = 220$

For the first cell there were 30 adolescents from the non-fluoridated area with caries. However, the expected number was 24.55, giving:

$$\frac{(O-E)^2}{E} = \frac{(30-24.545)^2}{24.545} = 1.212$$

Performing this calculation for all four cells and adding these values together gives:

$$\chi^2 = 1.212 + 0.394 + 1.010 + 0.329 = 2.945$$

Contingency Tables: General Use of the Chi-Squared Test

In Example 12.5 (p. 102):

Let

n_1 = number of children receiving halothane
n_2 = number of children receiving incremental sevoflurane
n_3 = number of children receiving 8% sevoflurane
r_1 = number of children with an arrhythmia
r_2 = number of children not experiencing an arrhythmia
N = total number of children (see Table A.4).

The null hypothesis is that in the population of children having dental extractions under general anesthesia the proportion of children experiencing arrhythmias is the same, irrespective of the anesthetic used in the extraction. This common proportion is estimated by $\frac{r_1}{N}$. So

TABLE A.4 Incidence of arrhythmia under anesthetic

	Halothane	*Incremental sevoflurane*	*8% sevoflurane*	*Total*
Any arrhythmia	24	4	8	$r_1 = 36$
No arrhythmias	26	46	42	$r_2 = 114$
Total	$n_1 = 50$	$n_2 = 50$	$n_3 = 50$	$N = 150$

the expected number of children having halothane and experiencing arrhythmia is estimated by $n_1 \times \frac{r_1}{N} = 50 \times \frac{36}{150} = 12$. The expected number (E) in each of the other cells of the table can be calculated similarly.

For the first cell 24 children were observed, whereas 12 were expected, giving:

$$\frac{(O-E)^2}{E} = \frac{(24-12)^2}{12} = 12.0$$

For assessing whether the chi-squared test is appropriate here, note that the minimum expected value (equal for the three cells in the top row) is 12.0, which is much greater than the generally recommended threshold of 5. Adding up for all 6 cells in the same way gives:

$$\chi^2 = 12.0 + 5.333 + 1.333 + 3.789 + 1.684 + 0.421 \approx 24.56$$

13: COMPARING SEVERAL MEANS

Examining Pairs of Groups Following a Multi-Sample Hypothesis Test

Let p be the probability of finding evidence against a correct null hypothesis for a single hypothesis test. Then the probability of obtaining no evidence against the null hypothesis is $(1 - p)$. For two such null hypotheses, the probability of finding no evidence against either hypothesis is given by $(1 - p) \times (1 - p)$. With three such null hypotheses, the probability of finding no evidence against any of the hypotheses is equal to $(1 - p) \times (1 - p) \times (1 - p)$. In general, for n correct null hypotheses, the probability of finding no evidence against any of them is $(1 - p)$ multiplied by itself n times or $(1 - p)^n$. Hence, the probability of finding evidence against at least one of the null hypotheses is given by $1 - (1 - p)^n$.

In Example 13.3 there are $n = 10$ pairings, and $p = P = 0.05$. The population means for the groups are assumed to be equal. Hence, the probability of finding evidence against at least one of the 10 pairwise null hypotheses is:

$$1 - (1 - p)^n = 1 - (1 - 0.05)^{10} = 1 - (0.95)^{10} = 1 - 0.5987$$
$$= 0.4013 \text{ or around } 0.4.$$

This probability has a similar order of magnitude to the approximate value of 0.5 given in the text.

TABLE A.5 Decisions of two dentists as to whether or not patients required treatment

	Dentist B		
Dentist A	*Yes*	*No*	*Total*
Yes	40	5	45
No	25	30	55
Total	65	35	100

Exact Probability of Evidence Against at Least One of the Pairwise Null Hypotheses (Bonferroni Correction)

Applying the Bonferroni correction to Example 13.4 sets the probability of finding evidence against a correct null hypothesis for a specific pair of groups at p = 0.005. The exact probability of finding evidence against at least one of the 10 pairwise null hypotheses is therefore:

$1 - (1 - p)^n = 1 - (1 - 0.005)^{10} = 1 - (0.995)^{10} = 1 - 0.9511$
$= 0.0489$, which is slightly less than the intended value of 0.05.

14: REGRESSION, CORRELATION, AND AGREEMENT

Consider the data in Example 14.5 (see p. 125; Table A.5).

The observed proportion of agreement is (40 + 30)/100 = 0.7. However, some of this agreement could have been expected by chance, and this is calculated from the row and column totals:

Under chance agreement, the expected number of cases in the "yes/yes" cell of the table is given by $\frac{65 \times 45}{100}$ or 29.25. The expected number of cases in the "no/no" cell is given by $\frac{35 \times 55}{100}$ or 19.25. The total number of expected agreeing cases is therefore 29.25 + 19.25 or 48.5. The expected proportion of agreement is therefore 48.5/100 or 0.485. Hence:

$$\kappa = \frac{0.7 - 0.485}{1 - 0.485} = 0.42$$

Solutions to Exercises

CHAPTER 1

1 Variables are:
  (i) Binary
  (ii) Continuous quantitative
  (iii) Whole number quantitative
  (iv) Nominal
  (v) Ordered.

2 The categories "no treatment," "filling," and "extraction" could be viewed as nominal in terms of different types of operation. However, in terms of the pain experienced by patients, there is an ordering of pain with extraction being the most painful procedure.

3 Any two of the following:
  (a) Understanding papers in journals: Insight into statistical methods used. Keeping up to date with advances in dentistry.
  (b) Clinical audit: Evaluation of new methods of treatment in dental practice and summary of practice records.
  (c) Health services research: Your dental practice could be involved in a large study along with several other practices. Insight into what the study team may require from your practice.

CHAPTER 2

1 Data set entries:
  (i) "99" indicates a missing value.
  (ii) "Six fillings" is a plausible entry.
  (iii) SOLAR is a string entry that was probably intended to be MOLAR.
  (iv) The age given is an error (the woman is now aged 35).
  (v) Making two visits in the last year is plausible.

  Note that plausible information is not necessarily correct.

2 The requirement for ethical approval gives both the researchers and the funding organization some protection. It enables the funding

organization's ethical experts to scrutinize the proposal and point out potential difficulties in the design that may have gone unnoticed by the research team. Avoiding patient distress is extremely important; good practice from an ethical point of view helps to achieve this. If things go wrong the result could be costly litigation. This can bring negative publicity to the research team and perhaps also to the funding body that made the research possible.

3 Some of the ways by which bias can arise in a community study:
   (a) Selection of the sample
   (b) Non-response due to absence
   (c) Non-response due to refusal to participate
   (d) Recall error
   (e) Differences between interviewers in recording responses
   (f) Misunderstanding of question because English is not first language.

   Some solutions:
   (a) Use a sampling frame that represents most (ideally all) of the community, e.g., electoral register rather than telephone directory.
   (b) For home-based interviews contact people when they are likely to be at home (e.g., in the evening) but not so late that some may refuse to answer the door.
   (c) Try to be as persuasive as possible!
   (d) If practical, use pain diaries (for instance) rather than rely on the imperfect memory of respondents.
   (e) Interviewer training – pairs of interviewers could rate some cases together.
   (f) Use multilingual interviewers or questionnaires in the language of the ethnic group.

4 A patient and public involvement group should be able to advise on some or all of the following:
   (a) Key concerns
   (b) The groups to be involved (e.g., older people, social organizations, dentists, health authorities)
   (c) Participant recruitment
   (d) Questionnaire items and interview topics
   (e) Lay summary for grant application
   (f) Participant information sheet and consent form
   (g) Data interpretation
   (h) Key individuals and organizations for dissemination.

This list is not intended to be exhaustive. Attention should be given to the national/cultural context.

CHAPTER 3

1 Type of study:
  (i) Cohort (patients would need to be followed up over many years)
  (ii) Cross-sectional
  (iii) Crossover (the same individuals could test the floss and tape over different periods of time)
  (iv) Case-control – as long as information on smoking can be obtained from either the dental notes or the patient.

2 For each case it would be virtually impossible to find a control having the same age *and* gender *and* socioeconomic group *and* ethnicity *and* practice. Fewer matching variables should therefore be used.

3 Student projects usually need to be completed in a matter of weeks or at the most months. Funds from an educational institution available to assist student project work are usually very limited. Cohort studies are generally conducted over much longer periods of time. They are expensive as dedicated project staff may be required.

CHAPTER 4

1 A simple random sample is one in which each member of the population from which the sample is taken has the same probability of being selected and every sample of a particular size has the same probability of being chosen. Such a sample is obtained by randomly selecting individuals from the complete population until a sample of the required size has been selected. For example, suppose that in a dental practice there are 1000 patients and a sample of 50 patients is required. The complete set of patients should be numbered consecutively from 1 to 1000. Next, 50 random numbers between 1 and 1000 should be obtained. The individuals having these numbers are then selected to make up the sample.

  A simple random sample may not necessarily be representative due to random fluctuation. For example, the proportion of women (say) in a small sample may be quite different from the proportion in the population.

2 Suppose that 20% of the patients arriving for an appointment are required for the sample. Before the clinic starts, a patient is selected

at random from the first five to arrive, and every fifth patient following the initial individual is then selected.

An advantage is that systematic sampling is readily accommodated in the daily routine of the receptionist. For example, every fifth patient in the appointment book could be highlighted to remind the receptionist or dentist to ask the patient about involvement in the study. Random sampling will produce an unpredictable pattern of patients to be asked and it is more likely that a patient will be overlooked.

A disadvantage is that with systematic sampling there is potential for sampling bias. For example, if the patients selected are those who have their appointment "on the hour," it is conceivable that most of them could be people in paid employment who prefer an easily remembered time to fit into their work schedule for the day.

3 Names listed in a telephone directory do not form a complete list of the population. People on low incomes are less likely to have a telephone so they will be under-represented. Individuals may be able to opt out of being listed, and these often affluent people cannot be included in the sample. For most families only one member is listed against the appropriate telephone number (typically an adult male). Women and children will therefore be under-represented.

CHAPTER 5

A Better Mouth Rinse: Case Study

1 The Xellent and Ynot groups might not be comparable because of differences between the two dentists (male vs. female, experienced vs. less experienced), practice locations (affluent vs. deprived), and types of patient (private vs. NHS). In addition, other factors may have changed over the five years, e.g., daily sugar consumption, use of chewing gum. Patients in the Xellent and Ynot groups should be as comparable as possible.

2 On the surface, this suggestion (systematic sampling) sounds very sensible. In its favor, it is likely to reduce the cluster effect of families coming to see Mary for treatment in consecutive appointments. Only one member of the family is likely to be chosen. Statistical methods generally assume that patients are independent of each other in terms of their characteristics. This might not be the case with family members. All patients from a particular family might have a clear preference for Ynot, perhaps due to a similar diet.

However, there are major pitfalls. Assuming that all slots are taken, there will be a maximum of eight patients recruited per day, or 80 over two weeks. This is well below the 100 per group advised by Peter. In addition, individuals who make appointments on the hour or half-hour could differ from other patients in important respects (they might, for instance, be more likely to be in paid employment). Unless she is extremely careful, Joan might overlook patients who should be included in the study. These selection biases could yield results that are unrepresentative of the practice patients in general.

The suggestion is also dubious from an ethical point of view (see Chapter 6), as the study will probably fail to yield useful results due to its small sample size and hence be a waste of resources.

Further Comments:
It might be worth offering Joan a supplement to her regular salary to take account of her additional responsibilities. If she is enthusiastic about the study, it is likely that she will be able to persuade more of the patients to participate. The study should not be extended beyond two weeks. If Joan gives in her notice, in three months' time Mary might be in the unenviable position of being without both a dental nurse and a receptionist.

3 This might appear to be a sensible idea as a crossover trial allows each patient to act as his or her own control; each patient is able to sample and respond to both mouth rinses. For most patients, the lapse of time between appointments will mean that there will be no memory of the effect of the first mouth rinse (carryover effect) by the time the second solution is used.

However, in practice a crossover design would be beset with problems. The study would have to run for a long time, as some patients might not return within a year. Other patients might never return. Hita would not be available to assist with the project throughout its entirety; changes in study staff can lead to biases.

4 Matching would be difficult to achieve. The process would be that if a patient were allocated to receive Xellent, the next patient with similar characteristics that arrives for treatment would be allocated to solution Ynot. For instance, suppose patients are matched for gender, age, and ethnic group. A white female aged 50 who receives Xellent would be matched with another white female aged between, say, 45 and 55 who receives Ynot (NB: Matching on age is usually done to within 5 or 10 years). This makes the groups comparable on the variables used for matching.

With "only" 45 patients per day there would probably not be many Indian females aged 70, for instance, to provide a match should one be required. Matching would make Joan's task far more difficult from an administrative point of view (remember that she threatened to give in her notice). On balance, matching would not be appropriate for this study.

5 This would be the preferred strategy. The study would be better if pink Ynot solution that looked identical to Xellent could be obtained – the trial could then be double blind. This means that patients would not know which mouth rinse they were receiving. Any preconceived patient biases about either mouth rinse would be avoided. If Hita organizes the filling of the glasses properly, Mary will be blind to the mouth rinse being given. Knowledge of the type of mouth rinse used might inadvertently lead Mary to make comments like "you'll feel better now" after a patient has used one particular brand, and thereby systematically influence the answers to the questionnaire for one of the two groups of patients (clinician bias).

   If by two months' time there is no sign of the pink Ynot solution appearing on the market, Mary has a dilemma. If she waits much longer, Hita will have left the dental practice before the study has been completed. If she starts the study immediately, it will not be double blind with the consequent biases. If it comes to this, it might be better to delay the study until Hita's replacement is in place.

6 Yes, it would be a good idea. Randomization of patients to groups (such as allocation by coin tossing) gives all patients the same probability (in this case ½) of being allocated to the Ynot group. There is then no allocation bias due to any of the practice staff. (NB: The study would then be a randomized controlled trial, the control treatment being the current mouth rinse, Xellent.)

   The treatment assignments should be made by someone not directly involved in the study (Peter would be ideal as he would have the resources to generate random numbers and hence a random sequence of heads and tails). He should then place the treatment assignments in sealed envelopes in the generated order. Mary should ensure that any unsuitable patients are excluded from the study (e.g., pre-school-age children). If a patient just about to enter the treatment room is both able and willing to be included in the study, Joan should open the next envelope in the series and the mouth rinse indicated should be given to that patient by Hita.

7 This is very poor practice. Hita presumably thinks that explaining the study to patients after the mouth rinse has been given will minimize the number of patients who refuse to complete the questionnaire. In fact, by doing this, patient resentment could be caused once the study has been explained. This might lead to a refusal to

participate any further in the study and extremely annoyed patients might change their dental practice.

Her suggestion is unethical, as all patients should give their informed consent following an explanation of the study, but prior to being entered.

It should also be explained that should they not wish to participate, they would receive the usual high standard of dental care from the practice staff. Most reasonable people would then be willing to oblige.

8 Patients should not be asked to complete the questionnaire at home. Nearly all of Mary's patients should be well enough to complete a simple questionnaire following treatment. The wishes of those who feel unable to do so should be respected.

It is generally accepted that postal surveys can have relatively low response rates (see Chapter 4). Patients might, for instance, lose their questionnaire. Joan would probably be unwilling to telephone patients, reminding them to return their completed questionnaires (this might increase the response rate but not solve the problem altogether). The non-responders are likely to be a serious source of bias as they will probably not be representative of the individuals who entered the study. They may, for instance, have "busy" lives and not be too concerned about details of their dental care.

9 Yes – this needs to be discussed between Mary, Joan, and Hita. Children are likely to be attracted to Mary's dental practice in considerable numbers because of her interest in anxiety reduction and, for the younger children, because of the toys available.

A tricky ethical issue concerns the autonomy of the child. Since the mouth rinse does not represent essential treatment, the child should be allowed to give personal consent rather than the parent(s) giving their assent. Some parents may not agree with this view. Young children (less than seven years?) may need to be excluded from the study, as the questionnaire may not be understood by them. However, if (for example) a six-year-old boy observes his sister completing a questionnaire following treatment he may wish to be included. In that situation, it would probably be best all round to allow him to do so. Considerable tact needs to be exercised by Joan.

10 Yes, indeed. The study is unlikely to be totally representative of the patients on her list. Those who come to the practice during the fairly short period of the study are likely to be patients who attend regularly and those undergoing a course of treatment that requires, for example, weekly visits to the practice. Those who attend only when in pain are unlikely to be seen during this short timeframe.

Young children and possibly the very elderly are unlikely to be included in the study due to the nature of the patient-satisfaction questionnaire. Those who decline to enter the study may be atypical of the patients as a whole. The overall findings must therefore be interpreted with caution.

11 Absolutely right! Mary's patients will be highly unrepresentative of the local community. Few of her patients will be Black Caribbean as 90% of her patients describe themselves as white. Those who travel to the practice from the suburbs are more likely to be affluent than the local residents. The position of the practice at first-floor level will deter the disabled (there will probably be many that are physically challenged locally, in view of the percentage receiving disability allowance). She might well attract a disproportionate number of anxious patients and children because of her approach to treatment and the presence of toys in the treatment room.

12 This decision would require careful consideration. The difference in satisfaction rates (85% vs. 65%) might be of clinical importance and statistical significance (Peter would have to check this). Patients may view the type of mouth rinse used as a minor detail and be justifiably more concerned about the effectiveness, cost, and pain involved in treatment. The costs of the two solutions should be compared in coming to a decision, and whether any patients have allergic reactions to Ynot. On balance further investigation might be worthwhile.

CHAPTER 6

1 Type of consent:
   (i) Passive (consent is assumed unless the class teacher is notified otherwise)
   (ii) Positive (the patient gives consent there and then)
   (iii) No consent

2 Studies that are too small may fail to produce useful findings and so waste money. Studies that recruit more patients than required are costlier than they need be. In both situations more patients are at risk of receiving an inferior treatment than is necessary. Information about a suitable sample size may be obtained from a pilot study (see Chapter 2) or from a literature review of similar studies.

3 It is unethical to ask individuals for information that is not required for a study. Why should they disclose details that do not need to be known by the researchers? This is also wasting the time of all concerned.

CHAPTER 7

1 The main reasons are:
   (a) The variable being studied might only take whole number values whereas a Normal distribution can, in principle, take any value.
   (b) Sampling fluctuations mean that even if the population had an exact Normal distribution, the sample would not.
   (c) In the real world, exact Normal distributions do not exist – almost always there are some extremely high and/or low values recorded.

2 With a Normal distribution there would be a concentration of observations around the mid-point of the time interval (5.45 pm), leaving around this time being more likely than around 5.30 pm or 6 pm. Here, the dentist is as likely to leave between 5.30 pm and 5.40 pm as between 5.40 pm and 5.50 pm (say) so the Normal distribution would not provide an adequate fit to the observations.

3 The number of teeth possessed by an adult cannot exceed 32. However, if the number of teeth remaining takes a Normal distribution, 95% of the observations should have values within two standard deviations (2 × 4) of the mean (30), i.e., between 22 and 38 teeth. This creates a contradiction, leading to the conclusion that the distribution has a large standard deviation due to a few small values. In other words, it is negatively skewed, not Normal.

CHAPTER 8

1 Individuals may or may not genuinely have dental caries; when checked by a dentist using a dental probe they may or may not appear to have caries. Misclassifications can occur in both directions (cases with caries can have a negative probe result and individuals without caries can have a positive probe result – probe results are checked against the definitive bite-wing radiograph). The positive predictive value (PPV) of a positive screening result (as a percentage) is given by:

$$\text{PPV} = \frac{\text{number with a positive screening result (dental probe) who have dental caries}}{\text{number with a positive screening result}} \times 100\%$$

   In other words, the percentage of those with a positive screening (dental probe) result who have dental caries.

2 If unaffected individuals must never receive a positive screening

result, unless there is little or no overlap of the two distributions (affected individuals, unaffected individuals), a high percentage of affected individuals will not be detected by the test (i.e., there will be low sensitivity). Such a test is unlikely to be of practical use.

3 (i) A "gold standard" decision is based on the most accurate method available for assessing the malignancy of a lesion. In this study it is obtained by histopathology. Accuracy of the clinical assessment is judged against the gold standard decision.

(ii) Sensitivity =

$$\frac{\text{number of lesions malignant on histological exam and positive on clinical assessment}}{\text{number of lesions malignant on histological examination}}$$

Specificity =

$$\frac{\text{number of lesions benign on histological exam and negative on clinical assessment}}{\text{number of lesions benign on histological examination}}$$

(iii) sensitivity $= \frac{12}{13}$, specificity $= \frac{13}{30}$

(iv) The clinical assessment is excellent at identifying malignant lesions (high sensitivity) but poor at picking out lesions that are not malignant (low specificity). If this method of screening is used routinely, many patients will be referred for further unnecessary investigations.

4 (i) Sensitivity =

$$\frac{\text{the number of diseased people positive to the test}}{\text{total number of diseased people}}$$

Specificity =

$$\frac{\text{the number of disease-free people negative to the test}}{\text{total number of disease-free people}}$$

(ii) The sensitivity of the screening test is the proportion of individuals out of those with documented dental agenesis (DA) who self-reported DA. The specificity is the proportion of individuals out of those with no documented evidence of DA who reported the absence of DA.

(iii) For population screening, the positive predictive value of self-reported DA is the crucial measure. This is the proportion of individuals out of those who self-reported DA who do have documented evidence of DA. For a prevalence of DA as low as 7%, even with high test specificity false positives may well outnumber the true positives, implying a positive predictive value of less than 50%. In this situation, self-reported DA would have little value as a screening tool.

CHAPTER 9

1 The standard deviation is a measure of the variation in the individual observations drawn from a population and is not influenced by the size of the sample. The standard error measures the degree of variation in the means of samples repeatedly drawn from the population. It is usually smaller than the standard deviation (put another way, the means of the different samples are similar) since large and small values within a sample tend to cancel each other out. The standard error decreases as sample size increases because of this cancellation effect.

2 Paired data occur where each observation in one set of data is associated with just one observation in a second set of data, e.g., dmft scores calculated on the same children at five years and seven years of age.

3 (i) With 95% confidence the true mean increase in the sales of this brand of mouthwash is between 2.5 and 9.5 bottles per week. The confidence interval is quite wide; 2.5 bottles per week is a modest increase whereas 9.5 is probably substantial.

  (ii) We have no information about the effect of the mouthwash on the dental health of those who start to use it. Economic considerations of whether a reduction of 10% in the price will lead to greater profits will probably be of more importance to the head office management of the chemist stores.

CHAPTER 10

1 A null hypothesis relates to a population, not to a sample. Also, this hypothesis should state a particular value for the mean in the population. The statement "is significantly different from" is therefore incorrect (such a statement might possibly be made about a sample). A more suitable null hypothesis would be "for the population of general dental practitioners in New York the mean number of patients treated per day is equal to 40."

2 If the *P*-value is very small, there is indeed strong evidence against the null hypothesis. However, if it is relatively large this indicates

weak evidence against the null hypothesis, which is not the same as positive support for it (this is illustrated by Example 10.2).

3 In the traditional interpretation of the *P*-value, 0.05 is the most commonly used benchmark, below which the null hypothesis is regarded as false (often described as rejection) and above which the null hypothesis is regarded as true (often described as acceptance). In the strength of evidence interpretation, 0.05 is one of a range of values that indicate moderate evidence against the null hypothesis, others being, say, 0.04 or 0.055.

4 When the *P*-value is equal to 1, the sample mean is equal to the null hypothesis value of the mean. Since the confidence interval is symmetrical around the sample mean, the null hypothesis value here will also be at the center of the confidence interval.

CHAPTER 11

1 Strong evidence against the null hypothesis occurs when a small *P*-value is obtained from an appropriate statistical test. With clinical significance the issue is whether the size of difference between groups is important from a clinical point of view, in that it would be sufficiently large to lead to a change in clinical practice.

Consider a comparison of two types of toothpaste, with groups compared on the mean number of fillings required during the study period. Strong evidence against the null hypothesis could occur without clinical significance if thousands of individuals were recruited. The difference between the means might be too small to be of clinical interest but due to the large sample size it could still be associated with a small *P*-value. On the other hand, if the study was small the difference between the two groups might be large enough to be of clinical significance, but the relatively large *P*-value that might be obtained from the test would indicate only weak evidence against the null hypothesis. Given that the true size of the difference is the crucial piece of information, the concept of clinical significance is preferred.

2 (i) For the population of dental practice patients in northwest England undergoing a procedure following a failed restoration, the mean time taken to perform the procedure is equal in the repair and replacement groups.

(ii) The *P*-value is the probability of obtaining two samples with a difference in mean procedure time between the two groups at least as great as that observed with the study samples assuming that the null hypothesis is true. In this case it is the probability of a difference between sample means of at least (25.15 – 21.65) or 3.5 minutes, both directions of the difference being of interest (the repair mean being greater than the replacement mean is of equal interest to the replacement mean being greater than the repair mean). The *P*-value measures the strength of evidence against the null hypothesis; a *P*-value of 0.044 indicates at least some evidence against the null hypothesis. There is evidence to suggest that the mean procedure time differs between the two groups. A confidence interval for the difference between the mean procedure times would give a range of plausible values for the difference in the population.

3 (i) For the population of dental hospital outpatients aged 18–70 years in Chennai, India, the mean MDAS score is equal for males and females.

(ii) With 95% confidence, the population mean MDAS score for females minus mean MDAS score for males could be as little as 0.5 or it could be as much as 1.5. Since the confidence interval does not contain the null hypothesis value of zero there is evidence against the null hypothesis (or one can reject the null hypothesis). Note that $P < 0.001$, which is very small, and relative to the width of the confidence interval, the lower limit of the 95% confidence interval is clearly separated from zero. On average, females are more anxious about dental treatment than males. The differences represented by the 95% confidence interval are unlikely to be of clinical importance; one unit on the MDAS might not represent a large degree of additional anxiety.

CHAPTER 12

1 The number of degrees of freedom is one less than the number of rows multiplied by one less than the number of columns = 2 × 3 = 6.

2 The correct confidence intervals are:

(i) e – values in the confidence interval are negative so female percentage is greater.

(ii) c – all values are positive and greater than the minimum difference of clinical importance (5%).

(iii) a – the null hypothesis value (0%) is just inside the confidence interval.

(iv) d – all differences in percentages are between –5% and 5% so none is of clinical importance.

(v) a – the null hypothesis value (0%) is inside the confidence interval and so is plausible.

3 (i) For the population of dentists in Iowa, the percentage accepting new Medicaid patients into their practice is equal for those who are metropolitan residents and those who are non-metropolitan residents.

(ii) With 95% confidence, the population percentage of non-metropolitan dentists accepting new Medicaid patients minus the percentage of metropolitan dentists accepting new Medicaid patients could be as little as 1.4% or as great as 16.8%. Since the confidence interval does not contain zero there is evidence against the null hypothesis (or "one can reject the null hypothesis"). The percentage accepting new Medicaid patients is greater in the non-metropolitan group. The differences at the lower end of the 95% confidence interval are probably not of importance in terms of dental health service delivery. The confidence interval is fairly close to zero so the evidence against the null hypothesis is not particularly strong.

CHAPTER 13

1 The assumptions most obviously untrue are as follows:

(i) The population variances are equal. The largest standard deviation divided by the smallest standard deviation is equal to 40. The ratio of sample variances is therefore extremely high at 40 × 40 = 1600.

(ii) Each sample is representative of its population. Children attending a dental hospital are likely to have different levels of usage for toothpaste and floss compared to children in the overall community.

(iii) Observations in each population follow a Normal distribution. The inclusion of the non-smokers will create a peak at zero; a Normal distribution is symmetrical around the mean.

(iv) Observations in one sample are independent of observations in the others. In general, groups are not independent for repeated measurements on the same individuals.

(v) Within each sample observations are independent of each other. Family members tend to have similar habits in terms of diet and dental hygiene.

2 (i) For the population of patients aged less than 21 attending this dental hospital, the mean age is equal in the three groups of patients (with family member, with friend, alone).

(ii) The P-value is the probability of obtaining samples with differences in mean age between the three groups at least as great as those observed in this sample, assuming that the null hypothesis is true. The P-value measures the strength of evidence against the null hypothesis; a P-value of less than 0.001 indicates strong evidence against the null hypothesis. It appears that patients attending with a family member are much younger on average compared to those in the other two groups.

(iii) Pairs of groups could be examined using the unpaired t-test. Note that the Bonferroni correction should be applied in interpreting the P-values from the pairwise analyses. Three pairwise comparisons are possible (family member vs. friend, family member vs. alone, friend vs. alone) so the appropriate P-value threshold is 0.05/3 or around 0.0167.

(iv) The age range for patients attending with a family member is likely to be wide whereas it is possible that there will be no patients under 18 attending alone. In such a situation, the "alone" group will have a much smaller variation in age. It is therefore questionable to assume that the three groups have the same population variance.

CHAPTER 14

1 The most likely values for Pearson's correlation coefficient are:

(i) a
(ii) e
(iii) b
(iv) c
(v) d

(See Figure 14.2, p. 121 for illustrations of these relationships.)

2 Association between two variables is where the values of one variable are, on average, related to the values of another variable. For instance, in a community a high daily sugar intake may be associated with a high DMFT score. Two variables may be associated through a third variable that may influence both of them and this can lead to spurious associations. For instance, in some developing countries, individuals receiving a high level of education may turn from traditional to Western (high sugar) diets. Sugar intake will be associated with DMFT score and level of education. However, it would be ridiculous to suggest the causal relationship that learning assists the development of caries!

3 If two raters are assessing patients, the vast majority of whom are thought to belong to one of the two categories, e.g., if 95% of a series of patients are thought to have healthy teeth with just 5% having decayed teeth, two dentists will agree on around 90% of the cases (actually $0.95 \times 0.95 + 0.05 \times 0.05$ or 90.5%) by chance.

4 (i) For the population of schools in North Carolina, the regression coefficient (slope) for the proportion of kindergarten children in the school with one or more decayed primary teeth (prop dt) against the proportion of children in the whole school enrolled for free or reduced-price school meals (prop FRSM) is equal to zero. (Equivalently, for this population the correlation between the proportion of children in the whole school enrolled for free or reduced-price school meals and the proportion of kindergarten children in the school with one or more decayed primary teeth is equal to zero.)

(ii) In practice, a high proportion of children enrolled for free or reduced-price school meals, indicating a high level of poverty, might be linked with a higher proportion of young children with evidence of decay in their teeth. In poorer areas the level of dental health provision might be lower as it is known that many dentists prefer to work in more prosperous districts. People living in deprived areas may have less money to spend on products related to dental hygiene and might see dental health as a lower priority than, say, having sufficient food in the house.

(iii) The value 0.0305 is the slope of the regression line. This indicates the expected increase in the proportion of kindergarten children in the school with one or more decayed teeth if the proportion enrolled for free or reduced-price school meals is increased by 1 (it is more meaningful to state that 0.00305 is the increase if the proportion having free or reduced-price school meals is increased by 0.1).

(iv) With 95% confidence, the population value for the slope could be as little as 0.001 or as great as 0.0604. Since the confidence interval does not contain zero, there is evidence against the null hypothesis. However, the lower limit of the 95% confidence interval is so tiny that, were this to be the true value, the finding would not be of practical importance.

(v) These findings do not necessarily indicate that there is a cause and effect relationship between low household income and tooth decay in kindergarten children. This association could arise because of a third variable related to both low household income and tooth decay that provides the true explanation.

CHAPTER 15

1 The data contain negative values, for which logarithms do not exist. Hence it would be impossible to analyze the transformed data.
2 The distribution of DMFT scores is generally skewed, with a few very high values. A test that does not require the assumption of Normality is appropriate, e.g., the Wilcoxon two-sample test for two independent groups. Samples need to be representative of the population of young adults in London and Edinburgh. DMFT scores need to be assessed in the same way in the two cities (preferably by the same examiner(s)).
3 Any set in which the lowest observation is less than a particular value and the highest observation is greater than a certain value, e.g., < 5, 6, 9, 12, 16, > 18.
4 The scatter diagram should have a downwards slope overall as the correlation is negative. For Spearman's rank correlation to be close to perfect, most of the lines joining adjacent points (moving across horizontally) should have a negative gradient. For Pearson's correlation to be closer to zero, most of the points should lie away from any fitted straight line.

CHAPTER 16

1 A power of 0.5 implies that there is only a 50% chance that a true alternative hypothesis will be detected; this is an unacceptable risk.
2 The difference between the means is 5 – 3 = 2, so the standardized mean difference (divide the mean difference by the assumed standard deviation) is 1.0. The rule of 16 gives the estimated number per group as 16 divided by the square of the standardized mean difference or 16 (*Stata* gives the same answer).
3 If the power is set at 0.9, the rule of 21 gives a rough approximation for the number required in each group of 21 divided by the square of the standardized mean difference. Since 21 is more than 16, the rules show that greater power comes at the cost of a larger sample-size requirement.

CHAPTER 17

1. Some reasons as to why the journal article might not be identified by the database are:
   (a) The journal may not be indexed in the database.
   (b) The keywords used in the search are unable to identify the paper.
   (c) The paper may have only just been accepted for publication and not yet been added to the database.
   (d) The paper may have been published prior to the period covered by the database.
2. Of the 206 papers identified, there were no systematic reviews, meta-analyses, randomized controlled trials, or cohort studies. All the studies published in the journal during this period were therefore of low research quality.
3. Divide the studies into groups by the types of dentition covered: (A) primary dentition only, (B) permanent dentition only, (C) both types of dentition. Only Groups A and C would be included in the meta-analysis for primary dentition whereas only Groups B and C would be included in the meta-analysis for permanent dentition.

References

Abasaeed, R., A.M. Kranz, and G. Rozier. 2013. The Impact of the Great Recession on Untreated Dental Caries Among Kindergarten Students in North Carolina. *J Am Dent Assoc* 144: 1038–46.

Altman D.G., S.M. Gore, M.J. Gardner, and S.J. Pocock. 2000. Statistical Guidelines for Contributors to Medical Journals. In *Statistics with Confidence: Confidence Intervals and Statistical Guidelines*, edited by D.G. Altman, D. Machin, T.N. Bryant, and M.J. Gardner, pp. 171–90. London: BMJ Books.

Appukutton, D., S. Subramanian, A. Tadepalli, and L.K. Damodaran. 2015. Dental Anxiety Among Adults: An Epidemiological Study in South India. *N Am J Med Sci* 7: 13–18.

Armitage, P., G. Berry, and J.N.S. Matthews. 2001. *Statistical Methods in Medical Research* (4th ed.). Oxford: Blackwell.

Baelum, V., L.D. Nielsen, L.D. Greve, and S. Rølling. 2011. The Validity of Self-Reported Dental Agenesis. *Eur J Oral Sci* 119: 282–7.

Blayney, M.R., A.F. Malins, and G.M. Cooper. 1999. Cardiac Arrhythmias in Children During Outpatient General Anaesthesia for Dentistry: A Prospective Randomised Trial. *Lancet* 354: 1864–6.

Borzabadi-Farahani, A. and A. Borzabadi-Farahani. 2011. Agreement Between the Index of Complexity, Outcome, and Need and the Dental and Aesthetic Components of the Index of Orthodontic Treatment Need. *Am J Orthod Dentofacial Orthop*. 140: 233–8.

Chu, S.J. 2007. Range and Mean Distribution Frequency of Individual Tooth Width in the Maxillary Anterior Dentition. *Pract Proced Aesthet Dent* 19: 209–15.

Cohen, J. 1960. A Coefficient of Agreement for Nominal Scales. *Educ Psychol Meas* 20: 37–46.

Coles, E., K. Chan, J. Collins, G.M. Humphris, D. Richards, B. Williams, and R. Freeman. 2011. Decayed and Missing Teeth and Oral-health-related Factors: Predicting Depression in Homeless People. *J Psychosom Res* 71: 108–12.

Dawes, C. 2003. What Is the Critical pH and Why Does a Tooth Dissolve in Acid? *J Can Den Assoc* 69: 722–4.

Day, R.A. and B. Gastel. 2016. *How to Write and Publish a Scientific Paper* (8th ed.). Santa Barbara: ABC-CLIO.

De Gregorio, C., A. Arias, N. Navarrete, R. Cisneros, and N. Cohenca. 2015. Differences in Disinfection Protocols for Root Canal Treatments Between General Dentists and Endodontists. A Web-based Survey. *J Am Dent Assoc* 146: 536–43.

Fleiss, J.L., B. Leven, and M.C. Paik. 2003. *Statistical Methods for Rates and Proportions* (3rd ed.). New Jersey: Wiley.

Gomes, P.B., S.H. Ferreira, V.C. Poletto, J. Bervian, and P.F. Kramer. 2011. Bibliometric Evaluation of the Scientific Production of the *Stomatos Dental Journal. Stomatos* 17: 20–31.

Güneri, P., J.B. Epstein, A. Kaya, A. Veral, A. Kazandi, and H. Boyacioglu. 2011. The Utility of Toluidine Blue Staining and Brush Cytology as Adjuncts in the Clinical Examination of Suspicious Oral Mucosal Lesions. *Int J Oral Maxillofac Surg* 40: 155–61.

Hajivassiliou, E.C. and C.A. Hajivassiliou. 2015. Informed Consent in Primary Dental Care: Patients' Understanding and Satisfaction with the Consent Process. *Br Dent J* 219: 221–4.

Hayden, C., J.O. Bowler, S. Chambers, R. Freeman, G. Humphris, D. Richards, and J.E. Cecil. 2013. Obesity and Dental Caries in Children: A Systematic Review and Meta-analysis. *Community Dent Oral Epidemiol* 41: 289–308.

Heasman, P.A., L.E. Macpherson, S.A. Haining, and M. Breckons. 2015. Clinical Research in Primary Dental Care. *Br Dent J* 219: 159–63.

Herring, J. 2014. *Medical Law and Ethics* (5th ed.). Oxford: Oxford University Press.

Iheozor-Ejiofor, Z., H.V. Worthington, T. Walsh, L. O'Malley, J.E. Clarkson, R. Macey, R. Alam, P. Tugwell, V. Welch, and A.M. Glenny. 2015. Water Fluoridation for the Prevention of Dental Caries. *Cochrane Database Syst Rev.* CD010856. Doi: 10.1002/14651858.CD010856.pub2

Inchley, J., D. Currie, T. Young, O. Samdal, T. Torsheim, L. Augustson, F. Mathison, A. Aleman-Diaz, M. Molcho, M. Weber, and V. Barnekow. eds. 2016. *Growing up Unequal: Gender and Socioeconomic Differences in Young People's Health and Well-being. Health Behaviour in School-aged Children (HBSC) Study: International Report for the 2013/2014 Survey.* Copenhagen: WHO Regional Office for Europe (Health Policy for Children and Adolescents, No. 7).

Jackson, D., P.M.C. James, and F.D. Thomas. 1985. Fluoridation in Anglesey 1983: A Clinical Study of Dental Caries. *Br Dent J* 158: 45–9.

Javidi, H., M. Tickle, and V.R. Aggarwal. 2015. Repair vs Replacement of Failed Restorations in General Dental Practice: Factors Influencing Treatment Choices and Outcomes. *Br Dent J* 218: E2. Doi: 10.1038/sj.bdj.2014.1165.

Johnson, R.P. and B. Quinn. 2011. The Role of Clinical Audit in General Dental Practice. *Dental Nursing* 7: 464–8.

Joshi, A. 2004. An Investigation of Post-Operative Morbidity Following Chin Graft Surgery. *Br Dent J* 196: 215–18.

Jovanovic, B.D. and P.S. Levey. 1997. A Look at the Rule of Three. *Am Stat* 51: 137–9.

Kay, E.J., N. Ward, and D. Locker. 2003. A General Dental Practice Research Network: Philosophy, Activities and Participant Views. *Br Dent J* 194: 545–9.

Lambden, P. ed. 2002. *Dental Law and Ethics.* Oxford: Radcliffe Medical Press.

Lancaster, G.A., S. Dodd, and P.R. Williamson. 2004. Design and Analysis of Pilot Studies: Recommendations for Good Practice. *J Eval Clin Pract* 10: 307–12.

Landis, J.R. and G.G. Koch. 1977. The Measurement of Observer Agreement for Categorical Data. *Biometrics* 33: 159–74.

Leathard, A. and S. McLaren. eds. 2007. *Ethics: Contemporary Challenges in Health and Social Care.* Bristol: Policy Press.

Lee, K.J., R.L. Ettinger, H.J. Cowen, and D.J. Caplan. 2015. Health Trends in a Geriatric and Special Needs Clinic Patient Population. *Spec Care Dentist* 35: 303–11.

Lehr, R. 1992. Sixteen s Squared over d Squared: A Relation for Crude Sample Size Estimates. *Stat Med* 11: 1099–102.

Masood, M., Y. Masood, and J.T. Newton. 2015. The Clustering Effects of Surfaces Within the Tooth and Teeth Within Individuals. *J Dent Res* 94: 281–8.

Matsui, M., N. Chosa, Y. Shimoyama, K. Minami, S. Kimura, and M. Kishi. 2014. Effects of Tongue Cleaning on Bacterial Flora in Tongue Coating and Dental Plaque: A Crossover Study. *BMC Oral Health* 14: 4.

McKernan, S.C., J.C. Reynolds, E.T. Momany, R.A. Kuthy, E.T. Kateeb, N.B. Adrianse, and P.C. Damiano. 2015. The Relationship Between Altruistic Attitudes and Dentists' Medicaid Participation. *J Am Dent Assoc* 146: 34–41.

Memon, A., S. Godward, D. Williams, I. Siddique, and K. Al-Saleh. 2010. Dental x-rays and the Risk of Thyroid Cancer: A Case-control Study. *Acta Oncol* 49: 447–53.

Moraga, J. 2014. Levels of Evidence and Geographic Origin of Articles Published in Chilean Dental Journals. *J Oral Res* 3: 36–9.

Murray, J.J., C.R. Vernazza, and R.D. Holmes. 2015. Forty Years of National Surveys: An Overview of Children's Dental Health. *Br Dent J* 291: 281–5.

Nelson, T.M., J.H. Berg, J.F. Bell, P.J. Leggott, and A.L. Seminario. 2011. Assessing the Effectiveness of Text Messages as Appointment Reminders in a Pediatric Dental Setting. *JAMA* 142: 397–405.

Owen, J. 1898. A Series of Four Cases of Swallowing Artificial Teeth Treated in the Royal Southern Hospital, Liverpool during the Last Six Months. *J Br Dent Assoc* 19: 467–9.

Ozar, D.T. and D.J. Sokol. 2002. *Dental Ethics at Chairside: Professional Principles and Practical Applications* (2nd ed.). Washington, DC: Georgetown University Press.

Popper K. 1980. *The Logic of Scientific Discovery* (4th ed. revised). London: Hutchinson.

Porter, S. 2006. Strong Association Between Areca Nut Use and Oral Submucous Fibrosis: Is There Any Association Between Areca Nut Use and Oral Submucous? *Evid Based Dent* 7: 79–80.

Probst, J.C., S.B. Laditka, J.-Y. Wang, and A.O. Johnson. 2007. Effects of Residence and Race on Burden of Travel for Care: Cross Sectional Analysis of the 2001 US National Household Travel Survey. *BMC Health Serv Res* 7: 40.

Rattan, R., R. Chambers, and G. Wakeley. 2002. *Clinical Governance in General Practice*. Oxford: Radcliffe Medical Press.

Scheifele, C., A.M. Schmidt-Westhausen, T. Dietrich, and P.A. Reichart. 2004. The Sensitivity and Specificity of the Oral CDx Technique: Evaluation of 103 Cases. *Oral Oncol* 40: 824–8.

Scully, C. and S. Porter. 2000. ABC of Oral Health: Oral Cancer. *BMJ* 321: 97–100.

Skaret, E., P. Weinstein, P. Milgrom, T. Kaakko, and T. Getz. 2004. Factors Related to Severe Untreated Tooth Decay in Rural Adolescents: A Case-Control Study for Public Health Planning. *Int J Paediatr Dent* 14: 17–26.

Smeeton, N. 2002. Undergraduate Courses in Dental Statistics in Britain and Ireland. *Stat Educ Res J* 1: 45–8.

Sprent, P. and N.C. Smeeton. 2007. *Applied Nonparametric Statistical Methods* (4th ed.). Boca Raton: Chapman & Hall/CRC.

StataCorp. 2015. *Stata Statistical Software: Release 14.0.* College Station, TX: Stata Corporation.

Sterne, J.A.C. and G. Davey Smith. 2001. Sifting the Evidence: What's Wrong with Significance Tests? *BMJ* 322: 226–31.

Tanaka, S., M. Shinzawa, H. Tokumasu, K. Seto, S. Tanaka, and K. Kawakami. 2015. Secondhand Smoke and Incidence of Dental Caries in Deciduous Teeth among Children in Japan: Population Based Retrospective Cohort Study. *BMJ* 351: h5397.

Thabane, L., J. Ma, R. Chu, J. Cheng, A. Ismaila, L.P. Rios, R. Robson, M. Thabane, L. Giangregorio, and C.H. Goldsmith. 2010. A Tutorial on Pilot Studies: The What, Why and How. *BMC Med Res Methodol* 10: 1. www.biomedcentral.com/1471-2288/10/1.pdf.

Thomas, F.D., J.Y. Kassab, and B.M. Jones. 1995. Fluoridation in Anglesey 1993: A Clinical Study of Dental Caries in 5-year-old Children Who Had Experienced Sub-Optimal Fluoridation. *Br Dent J* 178: 55–9.

Tickle, M., L. O'Malley, P. Brocklehurst, A.-M. Glenny, T. Walsh, and S. Campbell. 2015. A National Survey of the Public's Views on Quality in Dental Care. *Br Dent J* 219: E1. doi:10.1038/sj.bdj.2015.595.

Toverud, G., S.B. Finn, G.J. Cox, C.F. Bodecker, and J.H. Shaw. 1952. *A Survey of the Literature of Dental Caries*. Washington, DC: National Academy of Sciences-National Research Council.

Williams, A.C., E.J. Bower, and J.T. Newton. 2004. Research in Primary Dental Care. Part 6: Data Analysis. *Br Dent J* 197: 67–73.

Yamalik, N., S.K. Nemli, E. Carrilho, S. Dianiskova, P. Melo, A. Lella, J. Trouillet, and V. Margvelashvili. 2015. Implementation of Evidence-based Dentistry into Practice: Analysis of Awareness, Perceptions and Attitudes of Dentists in the World Dental Federation-European Regional Organizational Zone. *Int Dent J* 65: 127–45.

Index